Doula in a Day

Partner Support for the Woman You Love
during childbirth

TARA K HOWE

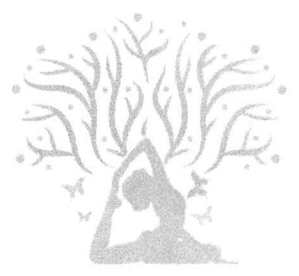

ISBN 978-1541273283

Printed in the United States of America
First Edition

Dedicated to all the mothers,
birthing partners and babies
I've had the honor of working with.
Thank you for sharing your worlds,
your wisdom and your lives with me.

And to all the new mothers, partners and babies
about to embark on this journey!

"When a doula is present during and after childbirth, women report greater satisfaction with their birth experience, make more positive assessments of their babies, have fewer cesareans and requests for medical intervention, and less postpartum depression."

DONA International

"Labor support by a minimally trained female friend or relative, selected by the mother-to-be, enhances the postpartum well-being of nulliparous mothers and their infants, and is a low-cost alternative to professional doulas."

Birth Journal

Table of Contents

Who is this guide for?

- Anyone who loves and values the woman giving birth.
- Anyone who will be an active part of the birth.
- Anyone who wants to better understand birth and how to be available during the perinatal period (around the time of birth) in a loving way.
- Mothers, Fathers, Partners, Families & Friends.

What is a doula?

A doula is someone who supports a woman through childbirth and the perinatal period. Traditionally and cross-culturally, groups of women have used their experience, compassion and networking to care for and support the laboring mother. Today, though times have changed, the needs of a laboring woman have not.

- Doulas SUPPORT mothers physically and emotionally during labor.

- Doulas ADVOCATE for the mother's choices and well-being.

- Doulas TRUST the mother's ability to birth.

Doulas DO NOT provide medical care

However, in today's highly medicalized system, doulas DO need to understand the medical environment and the realities behind the standard interventions in order to be able to do their jobs as advocates.

What is a doula?
A doula is YOU.

How to Use This Handbook

The handbook is relatively short so that you can read it from beginning to end in a day.

The importance of advocating for and supporting a woman during birth (which is so very individual for each woman) cannot be fully appreciated or achieved without understanding the *American Medical Model of Birth* and the *physiology and energetics of birth*.

The handbook is divided into three parts:

1. Understanding Birth
2. Being a Birth Doula
3. Postpartum Care

You will find a quick reference guide at the end to make the information readily accessible during labor.

Introduction

"Inside each of us is this seed of ancestral wisdom and natural intelligence – it is the mother matrix and it is within our DNA. Trust in women's inherent wisdom to instinctively and ecstatically give birth, and welcome the babies of the earth with deep love, warm hands, conscious intent, and gentle touch. This is the biggest gift we can give to humanity in the new millennium." www.birthemissary.com

I would like to write about birth in a way that honors the ultimate process of creation that it is. There is no one 'right' way to go about it. Each woman, each situation, each and every birth is unique. We look for cookie-cutter ways of describing and preparing for birth as though this could give us safe passage and no surprises along the journey. But that hope is to dishonor the very nature of creation, the very power of birth. We are animals and spirits both equally and importantly. It is wise to honor those innate aspects within. What I have learned from my own births, from attending the births of others as a doula and therapist, and my background as a student of biochemistry, anthropology and eco-psychology shapes a very different form of birth than the mechanistic medical model currently offered in the mainstream. And some of that view is what I hope to offer here.

It is a touchy subject, to speak about birth. It doesn't get any more personal than our views on life, sexuality and death; and all three are present during pregnancy and birth. That is also why we have the possibility of being transformed and re-birthed ourselves when we give birth or become a part of birth.

The process of birth has often been compared to the travel of the labyrinth. Many cultures celebrated this recognition through time, sometimes having clay tablets with labyrinths etched into them or drawings on the walls for the woman to follow during labor. In places where there is less focus on electrical monitors and technology for birth, the very essence of the journey is not forgotten; birth remains a passage.

A woman makes her way into the labyrinth and must also find her way out.

To walk with a woman through birth is to respect and allow for the unfolding of this passage.

As a doula/birth partner, you **do not** need to have all the answers.
You cannot have all the answers.
Nobody does.

You cannot be expected to 'fix' anything.
There is nothing to fix.

But there is a way of being that can be very helpful to a woman during birth. It is called 'holding space'.

Perhaps you will need to go through the readings and learn the techniques to come to a place where you feel like you can 'hold space', or perhaps it just takes your being there, fully present in the moment without judgment. No matter what your journey is to finding the capacity to 'hold space' for your partner or loved one, it is this one capacity—to hold space (Chapter 9)—that defines your ability to be of service to another in birth; and an incredible skill to accomplish.

Getting Started

"There is a secret in our culture, and it's not that childbirth is painful, it's that women are strong." Laurie Stavoe Harma

In America, hospital births are generally regarded as the safest births. As a culture, we tend to believe that the United States leads the world in its technological advances; implying better birth outcomes.[1] We rarely hear of mother and child deaths at birth, yet they not only still happen, maternal mortality (mothers dying around the time of birth) has been on the rise in the U.S.[2], and our infant mortality rates (babies dying around the time of birth) are higher than 41 other countries.[3]

Cesarian section rates, according to the World Health Organization, should be between 10-15% of total births.[4] Cesarian rates above fifteen percent increase the risk of death and complications for mother and child. In the United States, we have an average far above the guideline at 32.8%[5] (fluctuating between 7-70% depending on the hospital).[6]

Furthermore:
- Mothers who receive C-sections are 2.84 times more likely to die than those having a vaginal birth.[7]
- Risk of placenta accreta (severe obstetric complication where the placenta attaches deep within the abdominal cavity and can hemorrhage) increases with each subsequent c-section.[8]
- Low-risk babies born by cesarean were nearly three times more likely to die within the first month of life than those born vaginally.[9]
- Women receiving emergency c-sections were 6 times more likely to suffer from postpartum depression than those with spontaneous vaginal or forceps delivery.[10]
- Women who have c-sections are less likely to successfully breastfeed their children.[11]

As the statistics demonstrate, this single technological advance that was once used only in extreme circumstances is now over-utilized in a way that undermines the health, safety and emotional well-being of mother and child.

Yet the tendency towards technological intervention does not stop at cesarian section. Some of the most common medical lead to similarly poor results.

According to physician Marsden Wagner, episiotomies result in a "26% higher chance of a scar that requires suturing, 53% increased chance of having pain during sexual intercourse and two-fold increase to suffer fecal incontinence."[12] All this, despite the fact that episiotomies have NOT been shown to prevent tears or damage to the pelvic floor or damage to the baby in an extended labor (the most common stated reasons for giving episiotomies).[13]

Furthermore, 1/4 of women receiving epidurals will have complications:
 3 times greater chance of dying
 2 times greater chance of c-section
 1/500 chance of temporary paralysis
 1/500000 chance permanent paralysis

Additionally:
 10% of epidurals do not work at all
 1/3 of women who receive and epidural will have resulting back pain lasting one week to several months after labor
 8-12% of cases will lead to severe lack of oxygen for baby[14]

Ultrasound leads to an increase risk in preterm labor while simultaneously not being proven to improve perinatal outcomes in its use.[15]

The list goes on.

In the years I have spent as a doula, therapist and mother, the one thing that stands out to me is this: **It is not the lack of a woman's capacity to give birth that causes problems in labor, it is that women and their partners rarely expect what happens in the hospital setting and get caught in a series of interventions for which they are ill-prepared, leading to questionable outcomes.**

This book isn't about telling a woman whether to have a 'medicated' or 'unmedicated' birth or whether to birth in a hospital or at home, this book is about pointing out how poorly understood the process of birth has become in our everyday minds as women and partners preparing for birth. It is about understanding where common practices are problematic. Without an adequate understanding of our system and how it came to be, women and couples are generally ill-equipped to respond to the medical staff's insistence on protocol under the guise of 'safety' once in the hospital. One mom-to-be once said it best: "If I hadn't just been at my sister's birth, I would never, in a million years, have understood what to expect at my own son's birth and know how to make my choices."

In a comprehensive study on women's perceptions of labor published in 2006, the authors cite: "Our maternity care system is profoundly failing to provide care that many mothers told us they want and that is in the best interest of themselves and their babies."[16]

The elephant in the room here is the complete denial of the most fundamental element:

The Mother Gives Birth.

Not the doctor, the nurses, the midwife, the doula, or any technology in the room. The mother is the one, in a unique dance with her baby, who brings the child into the world. We must be able to trust her wisdom, her strength, her ability to transform and her ability to birth in order to fully support her through this process. A mother travels incredible terrain to birth a child, no matter which route she takes. Despite the technological advances, this intense process of transformation and strength cannot be underestimated or simply eliminated with the use of technology.

Each woman has a different sense of her body, her needs, and the place she will feel the safest for delivery. All of these elements are of critical importance when deciding where and how to birth.

No matter what her beliefs, it is helpful if the woman who is birthing understands the environment in which she will be birthing prior to giving birth so she knows what she is getting into and what her choices are. The promises being made by obstetricians ("I won't give you a c-section unless it is absolutely necessary) are not always what they seem, just as a midwife or doula who claims there is no potential risk in birth is not acknowledging reality. Additionally, unassisted birth has its own elements to consider. If a woman knows in advance the benefits and risks of each environment, she is more prepared for what will come. If she is prepared for what will come, and you have discussed these concerns and desires together, then you are more prepared as a doula to advocate and support this woman throughout the birth she chooses.

This book is divided into three parts to help you achieve your role:

PART I (UNDERSTANDING BIRTH) is a condensation of the incredible information available today in regards birth statistics, processes, and mother-centered birth.
PART II (BEING A DOULA) is a collection of techniques that are applicable to ALL birth situations, whether hospital, birth center, home birth or unassisted.
PART III (POSTPARTUM CARE) gives essential information on the postnatal period and your role as a doula during this time.

Whatever you have known of the woman you love prior to this time, prepare to learn even more and become witness to her deepest abilities. It is an amazing journey for all involved and an honor to be invited along this path

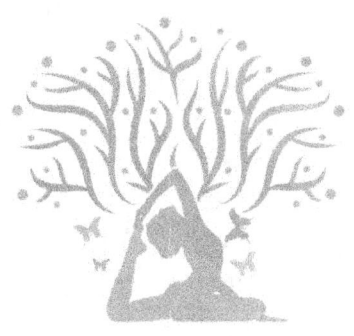

PART I: UNDERSTANDING BIRTH

1

Birth in the United States

"American maternity care, then, is under the control of tribal obstetrics. A small group, most of them men, are controlling birth in such a way as to preserve their own power and wealth while robbing women and families of control over one of the most important events in their lives." – Marsden Wagner, Born In The USA

MANY of the wealthy industrial countries that have lower infant and mother mortality rates than the United States ascribe to a midwifery model of care. Under the midwifery model of care, the process of birth itself is trusted and technology is used as needed rather than as the default method. Midwives are often the primary care givers during birth (whether in hospital or at home) and the obstetricians are available for emergencies and 'higher risk' pregnancies. In the Netherlands, for example, approximately 30% of deliveries occur at home and transfers to the hospital are relatively seamless, with respect amongst physicians, obstetricians, nurses and midwives for each other's skills and differences in knowledge.[17] In essence, the midwifery model of care is a *philosophy* not just practiced by the midwives themselves, but by all practitioners who ascribe to the idea that birth is a natural process to be supported, rather than feared.

The idea of the "midwifery model" of care in the United States is also known under a different name: "mother-centered" care. The Coalition for Improving Maternity Services (CIMS)[18] uses "mother centered" care to address these ideas, in part because the American history with midwives has been—with no excess drama attached for effect—a witch hunt. Studies surrounding well-trained midwifery care and the mother-centered approach demonstrate that mothers who are properly supported are more likely to have vaginal births, without complications and attach more profoundly to their children.[19]

Birth is a normal, natural and healthy process, and women and babies have the inherent wisdom necessary for birth.[20] Our bodies have developed a phenomenal system for birthing children over millennia of evolution.[21] Our birthing bodies are fascinating systems that can function in a wide-variety of circumstances and with highly effective methods of assimilating ALL the information at hand to find the best way forward through to the birth of the child. This is not something a machine can do. As you will see in Chapter 6: Labor Environment, the fundamental cocktail of hormones that come into play during an uninterrupted birth are an amazing testament to nature's most complex scientific mind and something we have not yet replicated in synthetic form.[22]

Given the sophisticated and natural process of birth and the effective mother-centered approach to childbirth in other developed nations, what happened in the United States to compel one-third of our nation's women to be drugged and cut?

The answer, like everything worth exploring, is not simple.

Prior to written history, artifact analysis shows that woman's ability to birth was revered.[23] With that being said, we also see evidence that other women assisted in birth.[24] Thus, the role of assisting a woman in birth began 'with woman'. This is one of the original meanings of 'midwife'.

First time mothers, especially, could benefit greatly from the help of other women with more experience while they learned to trust the process of childbirth within their own selves. Written references of midwives go back to Ancient Greece, the Bible and the earliest recordings of human history. Typically, the selfsame women (midwives) were healers and naturopaths and the caregivers for health in general.

The history of midwifery has its own complexities and it cannot be said that midwifery care (similar to current medical care) could prevent all infant or mother death. However, skilled and compassionate care during childbirth did increase the odds of healthy mothers and babies and could assuage some of the natural fear of childbirth.

But death remained a part of the birth process and so, when the European Barber Surgeon Guilds developed the use of forceps in the 1750s, there was a hope that more death could be prevented. Strangely, the barber surgeons themselves began as predominantly uneducated groups of men, generally butchers and barbers, who were completely unfamiliar with a woman's natural process in birth, but had access to tools that could be used to remove dead fetuses as needed. In the beginning, barber surgeons were only called into such cases. The transition from midwifery care to the barber surgeons, after the invention of the forceps, is one of the more strange and unsettling evolutions of control of birth that leads us to where we are today and worth further reading if you are interested. Because control over childbirth had such profitable potential, the guilds began to shut down the operations of midwives who were much better educated, experienced and prepared to assist women in labor.

This is immensely important in its implications: the process and skill in birth became devalued and the ability to save a single life through surgical tools took precedence.

In the end, this kind of surgical/forceps delivery lead to more complications and a higher death rate than that of the midwives. However, the poor outcomes went without notice for a long time, not only because of our fear of death and the hope that we might overcome even death itself, but because campaigns against midwifery and against women in general proved to be very effective.

Though the practice of midwifery was later revived in Europe and is strong in many European countries, the early 1900's in the United States showed a repeat of similar circumstances. In the colonial days of the American terrain, skilled midwives were a foundational part of the health care system, 'teaching in at least one university'[25] and having less infant and mother mortality than the physicians of the day.

However, early American doctors also knew:

Childbirth was an entry point to a thriving medical practice, often securing the woman's loyalty for her family's medical care [emphasis mine]. *In addition, obstetrics started gaining prestige as a medical specialty, whereas it was once deemed the 'most lowly' branch of medicine. In order to convince women to employ physicians rather than midwives, American physicians conducted a nationwide campaign against midwifery.*[26]

This concept remains true today. As a therapist and the previous Integrative Health Coordinator for a non-profit hospital, I am well-aware that 'getting women at birth' is a strategy to building the client base for a long-term, family-based medical practice. Convincing women that hospital birth is the safest birth also tends to ensure that all health-related concerns will be handled through the medical/pharmaceutical model[27] Which is not to say that those in medicine do not care or are out to deceive. Not at all. The practitioners I have had the honor to work with throughout the years care immensely. They want nothing but good outcomes for mothers, children and families. I am talking about the system of care that evolved, not the individuals within that system. We are each conditioned by our society and it is worth diving into the complexities that surround our ideas about birth so we can continue to create an environment that is optimal for women to birth.

Unfortunately, from the days of the barber surgeons onward, we got into a practice of intervening in birth not just during emergencies, but in general.

As a result, in a societal and subconscious way, we have come to devalue a woman's inherent wisdom in birth. And this is not just about the people outside looking in, this has happened for many women internally—the belief that she cannot do it without the doctor rather than the belief that the doctor (or midwife) is part of her team.

Robbie Davis-Floyd, a well-known medical anthropologist and birth culture expert, refers to our current birth practices as a 'technocratic model of birth'[28] in which the human body is compared to a machine:

> *"The male body is metaphorized as a better machine than the female body, because in form and function it is more machine like—more consistent and predictable, less subject to the vagaries of nature, and consequently less likely to break down ... Because of their extreme deviation from the male prototype, uniquely female anatomical features such as the uterus, ovaries, and breasts, and uniquely female biological processes such as menstruation, pregnancy and birth, and menopause are inherently subject to malfunction... As a number of physicians and medical anthropologists and sociologists have pointed out, our medical system has done a thorough job of convincing women of the defectiveness and dangers inherent in their specifically female functions."*[29]

In summary, Davis-Floyd explains why, when the female body is viewed as dysfunctional, birth is consequently perceived as one of the most extreme forms of malfunction. Since we have lived with these ideas for so long, many women have also come to believe this is true.

So why does this all matter?

The expectation that women's bodies are defective and that birth is pathological leads to an overall distrust in women and birth, which are two of the fundamental reasons we intervene in labor when it is not needed, creating all manner of difficulties, not only with the birth of her child(ren), but with her own sense of her ability to care for her child(ren) after birth.

Though there is a natural element to women's fears of pain, potential infant/maternal death and loss of control in childbirth, the extreme nature of these fears continue to persist in large part because women are not accurately informed of the risks, of the reasons interventions are performed, and because they are so often treated (and come to believe for themselves) as if they are not adequately equipped to give birth.

Since the dominant group controlling the perception of childbirth in the United States—as Marsden Wagner suggests in the opening quote of this chapter—is the American College of Obstetrics and Gynecology, we live with the idea that a technological birth is the safest birth.

Regrettably, as we have explored, many of the current day medical practices that espouse 'safety' as the reason for the standards of medical care disguise the true underlying causes. Ex. Labor induction is often called for under the false reason of infant/mother safety when, in fact, a significant number of inductions occur out of convenience for the physician's schedule.[30]

When women and families are not given the real reasons for the kind of care and interventions being prescribed to them, they are not truly able to make informed decisions about their care. And when a woman does not believe her body is capable of childbirth, we potentially strip from her one of the most fundamental wisdoms and sources of power that relates to bringing a child safely into this world and raising that child.

Once you understand this, the ability for you—as the doula—to better advocate for the woman you love increases exponentially. You will still need to discuss her wishes for birth, her fears in birth and the ways in which she wants you to be present during birth. But armed with the knowledge that her body is equipped to birth, and the history of the medicalized approach to childbirth, you and your partner can make decisions with a much deeper trust in your own authority.

2

The Medical Model

ONE OF THE biggest questions that plagued me as I attended the hospital births of other women was why there was this insistence on such a short timeframe in which to have the baby. From my own birth research and from the internal sense in my body that birth had its own rhythm that could be much longer (safely) than what hospital staff had been taught was safe, I felt that birth was an *unfolding* rather than a *production based* activity.

How on earth did all these incredibly intelligent and well-meaning health care providers come to believe that twelve hours was a standard timeframe for labor and that a textbook labor should proceed with dilation increasing at 1 cm per hour? We are not machines, we don't expect any other natural human function to occur with such prescribed timeframes, so why birth?

Finally, I read Jennifer Block's book, *Pushed: The Painful Truth About Childbirth and Modern Maternity Care,* where she speaks to the history of the current medical model of birth in the United States. She explains that this entire TIMED BIRTH element came out of experimental conditions that originated in the 1950's in Dublin, Ireland and was called "Active Management of Labor". I will give a condensed version below but her book is well worth the read.

Like many new laws or systems of practice, active management of labor originated in an effort to make one specific risky area of the birth process safer: prolonged labor. At the time it was developed, labor that went more than 48 hours was considered "prolonged." And a prolonged labor was one of the key risk factors for complications at birth.

At its experimental origins in Ireland, the cesarian section rate was 4%. Current American rates vary between 20-80%, and if you will recall, the risks for mother and child increase when c-section rates rise above 15%.

There is a generally accepted sense that about 5% of births will result in complications. That is no small number to be sure, but we also must remember that means 95% of births go on without an issue. However, in Dublin in the 1950's, they hoped to change even that 5%.

So, the doctors attempted to speed up birth that was prolonged (not all births, mind you). The theory was that a more active approach to labor would make it go faster, and it was assumed this would reduce the cesarian section rate and death rates.

They used synthetic oxytocin and amniotic rupture to increase the rate of contractions, BUT ONLY UNDER A VERY SPECIFIC SET OF CONDITIONS:

- MUST be a woman's first birth (called primigravida, statistics demonstrate that second births rarely go past 48 hours and mom's body is generally considered to have 'warmed itself into birth').

- Only women in <u>active labor</u> were admitted to the hospital (at least 4 cm and contractions lasting 15s-1m spaced no more than 5 minutes apart).
- A midwife or nurse was assigned to full-time care and observation of the woman (IE. She was never left alone with computer monitors).
- Labor that did not progress at a measured rate (1cm of cervical dilation per hour) was augmented by artificial oxytocin.[31]

And remember, this was still just a theory being tested, not an already validated experience being tested.

The outcome?

They were able to bring prolonged labors into a 24 hour window, but C-section rates ultimately INCREASED over the years of the study (from 4-9%) and there was a 12 fold increase in women requiring pain relief.[32] Though the goal had been to reduce the impacts of prolonged labor and the 4% c-section rate, it increased it.

Unfortunately, some physicians in the United States (also concerned with c-section rates that had tripled from 5-15%) began testing the method in the 1980's. The measured and controlled nature of active management also appealed to American physicians and the general managed and production based approach to life that continues to characterize the US. The American doctors, unfortunately, did not follow the Irish protocol–IE. Strict establishment of active labor, constant supervision, etc., instead taking a much more liberal approach to continued interventions.

In the end, c-section rates were <u>not</u> decreased in Dublin.

The following quote from Wagner summarizes the mentality of the American Obstetric mentality:

"Throughout the twentieth century, this arrogant belief that obstetricians know better than nature has led to a series of failed attempts to improve on biological and social evolution. Doctors replaced midwives in the United States for low-risk births, and the

later science proved that midwives were safe.... By embracing a medical model of birth and allowing obstetricians control of our maternity care, we Americans have accepted health care for women and babies that is not only below standard for wealthy countries but often amounts to neglect and abuse."

The principles of Active Management go through minute changes each year as different research and governing boards create new regulations, but the basic principles of active management (and therefore the medical model) have remained the same:

- Labor should be managed
- Cervical dilation should occur at 1cm/hour
- Interventions will be used to augment a labor that does not follow this rate
- Electronic fetal heart rate monitoring must be a part of the equation

Add these concepts to the already submissive and mechanized medical view of a woman's body, and the power, strength and wisdom of a woman in birth is all but forgotten.

Functional Outcomes of Active Management of Labor:

1. The definition of the normal upper limit to labor has been reduced from 36 hours (in the 1950s) to 24 hours in the (1960s) to 12 hours in 1972 when Active Management was introduced.
2. "Failure to progress" went from 3.8% in 1970 to 11.6% in 1989 and now accounts for ½ of cesarians for first time mothers.
3. Fetal distress rose from 1.2% in 1980 to 6.3% in 1989.[33]

What this means today is that we are utilizing a system that was originally only for the purpose of study, an exploration of a new methodology that was subsequently misapplied in the US even as the longer term studies showed the negative impacts.

This means labor in the medical model is conceived as a twelve hour process based on misinformation.

This faulty expectation, in addition to the way it fails to recognize the inherent wisdom of birth and imposes a regimented schedule on what is in fact a fluid process, is that it is also responsible for what we know as *The Cascade Effect.*

The Cascade Effect:

- The expectation for 12 hour labor leads to the increased use of pitocin, amniotic rupture and early admittance to hospital.
- Pitocin leads to levels of pain not experienced in regular labor.
- Need for pain relief, as the result of pitocin, leads to interventions that tend to slow labor and create further complications.
- Complications and delayed labor lead to an increased number of c-sections.

In the end, women are sometimes relieved they were in the hospital without realizing it is this very cascade effect generated by hospital protocol that contributed to the c-section: "Women are naturally grateful to the staff for the relief of their pain, not realizing that the staff exacerbated the pain in the first place."[34]

The World Health Organization, as we already covered, recommends c-section rates of NO MORE THAN 15%. Studies show that maternal mortality is significantly increased at rates above 15%. Though we have a wonderful ability to perform c-sections now in a manner much safer and less-intrusive than ever before—and this undoubtedly saves lives in the percentage of cases where it is truly a needed medical intervention—we have also created an environment more conducive to the occurrence of c-sections and other interventions without questioning the ethics of such an approach.

Unfortunately, just because you are aware of the risks inherent in the Medical Model, it does not make it easy to avoid interventions in a hospital birth. The entire birth culture is centered around the Active Management principles and it is difficult, if not impossible, for most hospital staff (doctors included) to work outside of this model even if they do see the problems with the model. Additionally, many physicians have never even seen an unmedicated birth or a home birth[35] which means many of our talented and educated specialists are completely unaware of the processes of uninterrupted birth.

The fundamental issue to come to terms with, then, is that our current medical model of birth is based on a study that failed in its goals yet became an entire philosophy of birth. It is an abuse of statistical data that leads to increased and problematic interventions rather than intimate process knowledge.

3

The Midwifery Model

"The medical model shows us pregnancy and birth through the perspective of technological society, and from men's eyes. Birthing women are thus objects upon whom certain procedures must be done. The alternative model…which I will call 'the midwifery model'…is a woman's perspective on birth, in which women are the subjects, the doers, the givers of birth." Barbara Katz Rothman

THE MIDWIFERY MODEL views birth as a normal physiological process rather than an illness, problem or disease to be 'fixed' wherein the woman and child are a team working together with the inherent wisdom to safely birth.

Principles of the midwifery model according to Robbie Davis-Floyd:
- Woman centered perspective.
- Defines women as active agents in pregnancy and birth.

- Female body as normal on its own terms.
- Pregnancy and birth as healthy, normal parts of women's lives.
- Holistic approach, defining body as an organism and an energy field in constant interaction with other energy fields.
- Viewing mind-body as one and mother and baby as an inseparable unit.
- Family rather than institution as the most significant social unit.
- The mother, not the practitioner, is the most significant birthing agent.

The midwifery model, it should be noted, is not only a model midwives can or do practice. Physicians can, and sometimes do, choose to proceed by more of this model. In contrast, some midwives may practice by more of a medical model.

Despite the still all-too-common belief that midwives are unskilled, they are, in fact, generally highly skilled and very knowledgeable and able to provide pre and post-natal care as well as many emergency services at birth. Depending on licensing and location, midwives can give medications, use Pitocin and IV's, suture, etc. Any of the books referenced in the bibliography will give an excellent overview of midwifery. And if you never have done this, try this for an exercise: Speak with a real midwife.

The reality is that most complications that arise do so with plenty of warning and well-trained midwives know how and when to transfer to the hospital. Evidence also shows, that so long as the hospital is not purposefully negligent in preparing staff for a c-section, transfer time for those living within twenty minutes of the hospital is equivalent to the amount of time it would take to prepare for a c-section in the same scenario WITHIN the hospital.[36]

The issue in the United States is the way in which the medical system does or does not work with midwives rather than the timing or the skill of the midwife. This stems back to perception and control.

In countries where there are skilled midwives and collaborative medical staff, home-hospital transfers are a matter of a phone call and preparation. Often midwives have hospital privileges and function in multiple locations (homes, hospitals and birth centers).

In countries where midwives are ostracized or deemed incompetent and treated with disdain or neglect, problems with transfer arise.[37]

Realize that the midwifery model of care does not say there is never a need for emergency services, but rather that this need is small and should be available WHEN it is needed.

The difference with the American maternity care system (medical model/active management) is that we treat every birth itself as if it is or will soon be an emergency. The implications and consequences of this conditioning will be more readily apparent as you read further into Chapter 7: Interventions and Chapter 6: Birth Environment.

Studies show the safest way for a low-risk woman to birth is with a midwife. Systems worldwide that combine the best of both models (medical and midwifery) have the lowest maternal and infant mortality rates and the highest levels of satisfaction and empowerment with the birth experience itself.[38] This also translates to other beneficial outcomes such as increased ability to breastfeed and better bonding and attachment between mother and child.

PAUSE—A Moment to Think

Are our bodies really machines? Is a woman's body inferior to a man's?

If you believe these sentiments, where do they come from? Are they yours or do they belong to the culture in which you live?

If you are a man, do you really believe your partner is inferior to you?

If you are a woman, do you really believe your body is defective or your female partner's body is defective?

In a Gaia philosophy of the earth, the earth has infinite wisdom and ability to provide homeostasis. Everything about the function of the earth is an incredibly designed system that evolves and meets the current demands placed upon it, balancing infinite ecosystems within. So it is with a woman's body.

Trust in the infinite wisdom of the woman's body and the years of evolution of this incredible form to birth a child.

What environments create that trust?

Quiet.

Dark.

Intimate.

Uninterrupted.

Safe.

Think of two of your most basic functions: the orgasm and the excretion of fecal matter.

Would you like someone to consistently monitor you, test your fluid levels and comment on how you are doing, finding 'pathology' in every aspect of your performance? Do you think, if it was this way, you might start to see yourself as defective? Do you think you could actually have a bowel movement or reach a peak orgasm if you are consistently monitored or being told you are doing it wrong?

Ina May Gaskin, renowned midwife, explains this with the Sphincter Law "which simply states that cervical, vaginal, and rectal sphincters work best in an atmosphere of privacy—for example, in a room with a locking door where interruption is unlikely or impossible. None of our sphincters can be commanded at will to open or relax, and once in the process of opening, they can close down again with fear or self-consciousness."[39]

The midwifery model of care—a mother-centered model of care—not only understands the process based phenomenon of birth but strives to include the best of the intuitive and scientific worlds. It is a model that exudes trust in the inherent wisdom in a woman's body, support for woman and child, and assistance/intervention where necessary; a philosophy that can be carried into any birth.

4

Unassisted Birth

Most people know that a woman can birth in the hospital or at home. Some know about an 'in-between' option called a Birth Center. However, there is a growing movement in the US towards unassisted childbirth, also sometimes termed 'free birth'. Rixa Freeze

UNASSISTED BIRTH simply means that a woman chooses to birth outside of the care of a physician or midwife. She may do it completely alone, with her partner or a doula present or with a midwife on call as back-up. But she chooses to take complete responsibility for the birth and the decisions she makes in regards the birth.

Though this may seem extreme to many, it raises some of the most fundamental questions about birth.

Rixa Freeze, an academic who has studied unassisted Birth at

19

length explains:

> *"This debate over safety goes beyond just words and ideas. It is a struggle over who, if anyone, should have the monopoly on defining which behaviors are appropriate and what are not. It is about social control and about how far our culture is willing to tolerate dissension and difference."*[40]

As a culture, we speak of safety as though a child coming into this world is the only factor. Mothers have greater incidence of post-partum depression with c-section and medicated births. The rate of maternal death in c-section is 4 TIMES that of a vaginal birth. Not bonding with your child is akin to a completely different kind of death that we never talk about and issues with breastfeeding are very common.

Whether people realize it or not, the strength that comes from birthing your child *in the way that is right to you* is a large part of what gives you the ability to care for your children in the best possible way.

'Free-birthers' know all too well what it means to speak out against the control element of mainstream birth, as a result, their questioning and forays into birth open up an important discussion about the process and control in birth itself worth examining.

Take a moment to ask yourself:

Where do you fit along the line of hospital-birth center-midwifery-free-birth?

How does your partner of loved one want to give birth?

Can you support her in this choice?

5

Understanding Labor

"When you yourself realize that you gave birth, not someone or something else–they didn't grow that baby, they didn't bring it down into the birth canal–you have a much more intense and personal relationship with that baby, and that's a basic feature of growing up as a whole healthy person." Robbie Davis-Floyd

IN THIS CHAPTER, I want to describe labor in a way that gives it the continuum and respect it deserves. Read it and understand it as the PROCESS that it is. When you read PART II: Being a Doula, techniques specific to each phase (with a quick review of the phases and what to look for) will be presented.

Labor is functionally divided into three phases:

1. First stage: Beginning of labor until the time to push (divided into

early & active labor & transition).

2. Second stage: Pushing through to birth.
3. Third Stage: Delivery of the placenta.

However, labor has an ebb & flow that goes beyond descriptions of first, second and third stage. What is really happening is that a woman's entire body is preparing to bring a baby into this world. This involves a complex system of interactions between the hormones, nerves, muscles, emotions and psychological and spiritual states, and everything a woman has learned and knows about her body and history.

The cervix—a combination of connective tissue and smooth muscle that both holds the baby in the uterus during pregnancy and then allows the baby access to the outside world during birth—makes an amazing transition over the course of labor.

The thick and closed cervix must thin (efface) and open (dilate) to allow the baby to pass. Throughout the stages that we call 'early' and 'active' labor, the baby goes through a series of rotations to descend the birth canal.

NOTE: A doula can help coach mother during labor by helping her focus on HOW she and BABY ARE WORKING WITH TOGETHER during labor.

Once transition occurs, the top of the uterus (the baby's home this whole time) needs to close down further around the baby before the urge to push is felt.

Even the urge to push and our current concept of 'pushing' has been called into scrutiny by a pioneering physician, Michel Odent who has been working with the importance of uninterrupted labor principles in France and finding a completely different picture of birth that emerges when women are not consistently monitored and interrupted.

REMEMBER: The process from a closed cervix to an open cervix and the descent and birthing of child (especially for first time moms whose bodies have never opened into this experience before) TAKES TIME!

This process of opening can take days to weeks to accomplish. The process, really, is occurring over the length of the entire pregnancy. The ability to grow and hold this child inside and then open and release the child into our arms is a single continuum with many beautiful transitions along the 10 month journey.

Unfortunately, as we saw in Chapter 2, the medical/active management expectations for labor is TWELVE HOURS.

One Mother's Story:

"Even by my third child, I was hard pressed to define an actual moment that labor began. Was it the two months prior that I had increasing pressure into my pubic bone and a sensation of increasing heaviness? Was it the slightly pleasurable twinges I had that reminded me my cervix was going through a process of slow opening? Was it after my husband and I made love and I got that feeling in my head of foggy dreaminess? Or a day later when I saw the acupuncturist and the fogginess increased with the same pressures I had been feeling for so long became just that much more? The contractions I had through the night that I called our midwife were full and good but not of an intensity I couldn't handle. By morning, my cervix had dilated to an '8'. Was this labor? For me, labor only 'began' when I had to surrender to pushing. That is when I really had to start working and letting go. Not pushing itself, but releasing into pushing, that 5 hour process, for me, was when labor began."

How and when to define the onset of labor is part of what shapes the expectation for length of labor.

These days, we use the terms 'early labor' and 'active labor' to give some division between an otherwise continuous process. In early labor, a woman is said to be having mild contractions, but still be able to breathe and talk through them, be of light countenance and doing ok with the world. For many women, this is true and day-to-day activities can be continued. However, as a doula, I have also seen women doubled over in pain during this phase. Our concepts of pain have so much to do with our own individual histories as well as our cultural perceptions. If we view birth instead as a labyrinth we are more able to honor that the difficult parts of the journey will be unique to each woman and unable to be measured by any standard.

A very concrete example of this, and something to bear in mind regardless, is the way many women who have suffered sexual abuse resist the opening of the cervix.[41] The opening of the cervix can pose an extreme threat for a woman who had to protect herself from the intrusion of a sexual abuser. The type of environment she needs to feel safe and the amount of time it might take her body to become accustomed to the strong sensations of labor in a way that is not threatening must be respected.

Through years of healing arts work, I have come to live by the adage that in healing *we cannot go too deep just too fast*. What this means is that a woman comes to each turn in the labyrinth of labor and must feel safe and able to open further into each new phase of the labor without being forced. She is literally entering whatever you call the cosmic version of death and transformation: she is becoming someone new in birth. It is important to note that many sexually abused women who birth vaginally experience a strong healing in the safe passage of their children when supported along this journey.

No matter what a woman's experience prior to birth, she is undergoing this radical transformation and will find her own rhythm when allowed to do so:

> *"During the birth of my daughter I felt immense power. Then I felt a feeling better than any orgasm I had ever had, as her sweet, slipper body left me. I immediately felt I'd do anything to feel that feeling again, that last moment of ecstasy. But by then I was caught in a wave of other ecstasies, the feeling of her warm body against mine, her soft purple skin turning pink in my arms."* [42]

A woman in a safe space can accomplish amazing things.

It is crucial to know that the first time we birth, the cervix itself goes through an enormous journey. It may take weeks for the cervix to become thin. This muscle has been responsible for holding a baby inside of a woman for nearly ten months. And prior to that time, the cervix remained in essentially the same configuration for the number of years this woman was alive. Imagine how long it takes to warm your muscles into a new activity. Say you are learning to pitch in baseball. After your first day, if you overdo it, you could be quite sore. In order to really learn to use this new grouping of muscles in any functional kind of way, it is going to take weeks. Mastering the motion is another thing altogether, but just getting the muscles into a new pattern of usage takes time and tends to involve discomfort. The same could be said for the cervix.

Defining the onset of labor, then, is quite difficult given these parameters, but absolutely crucial when we are within a birthing model that only 'allows for' a twelve hour window.

PHASES OF LABOR

ACTIVE AND EARLY LABOR

Active labor, the time that most physicians recommend a mother come into the hospital, is defined as:

- Contractions lasting for about 1 minute and occurring every 4-5 minutes.
- Cervical dilation of at least 4cm

In addition to this measured definition, many doulas, midwives and nurses will listen to the woman in labor as she speaks. If the laboring woman cannot finish a thought or a sentence while in a contraction, this is generally the sign that 'active' labor is well underway.

Early labor is essentially everything before active labor and you may never be able to quite pin-point where that occurs. The mucus plug could 'fall out' hours or weeks before contractions begin. The amniotic fluid (bag of waters) might break or leak in advance. Contractions could come in 20 minute intervals.

NOTE: Your physician or midwife will speak to you in advance about when to call during labor. And if you have any questions at all, call. This is YOUR birth team. You are not inconveniencing anyone.

This is what your team signed on for!

There is an unfortunate consequence of defining one part of labor as active and the other part early. It creates the expectation that only 'active' labor itself is ACTIVE or PRODUCTIVE. As should be clear by now, all labor (all pregnancy in fact should be considered some part of labor!) is active (accomplishing something).

Another issue with defining this stage of active labor is that it often creates a lot impending fear for a woman and her partner, because they are looking for a time that gets harder and bracing (as is natural to do with the expectation of pain) against this occurrence.

Labor generally progresses over a length of time in order for our bodies to physiologically adapt to the parts of the process. If you put your hand in a glass of ice water after just having had it in the sun, it will be shocking. But if you first put your hand in a glass that is lukewarm and slowly add ice, the perception of intensity is much less, though you will ultimately have your hand in the same cold water.

TRY THIS: Think of how it would feel if someone asked you to put your hand in this imaginary glass of water and told you they were going to add ice and that with each addition of the ice the glass would get a LOT colder. Before your body has even had a chance to process the experience itself, your mind is generating a response to this suggestion and a physiological process is already well underway. It is likely more uncomfortably colder because you have been told it is colder. At some point, had you not been told about the cold, you would ultimately feel it, but not only would you have adjusted substantially by then, you would not have been in psychological distress/expectation for that duration.

In the same way, then, active labor is not a defined moment and does not indicate a sudden onset of pain. Contractions do not necessarily go from easy to hard. This is a continuum.

TRANSITION

Transition is defined as the cervix dilating from 8-10 cm.

26

Transition, the way we speak of it in medicalized literature, online sites and most common media generates another level of immense fear in a woman. We are told this is the time that all hell breaks loose and we won't know what to do with ourselves. Again the reality is that being told to expect something tends to create just that scenario.

Elizabeth Davis, midwife and author of *Heart & Hands*, defines transition in a much more evolved manner:

> *"The mother is usually so immersed in her work that she hardly notices (others) comings and goings. To observe a woman at this time is a privilege; most have a softness about them as social masks fall away and deep beauty is revealed. Birth attendants must respect this phase of labor for what it is: a peak, out-of-body experience that prepares and rejuvenates the mother for the back-in-the-body, reentry phase of pushing and birthing. This changes dramatically with the 'I can't do this anymore' point near full dilation. It may be heralded by restlessness, complaining, shift in focus or loss of control."*[43]

This definition is much more appropriate and indicative of the intimate workings of the body. Physiologically, the changes in the body happen in a way that makes full and immediate integration of the intense sensations possible in quite the same way it is when a woman has contractions in active labor and finds the period of REST between contractions. However, surrendering into the time of transition occurs as a woman is allowed to sink fully into the intensity and may not last long at all. 'Transition,' as the name implies, is a form of transformation, of dying into one's own self and finding complete surrender to the process. It is an incredible moment and journey. It is not uncommon, either, for women to refer to desires to die or be afraid they might die, or break apart, etc. Be assured, we will not die or break apart and it is natural that a woman may feel these things! As you will find in Chapter 9, your role will be to simply support and be present so she can experience the transition.

I've seen too many women just at the end of transition, peaking to the point that the intensity is almost unbearable, and asking for pain relief, when just around the corner, the natural pain relief is about to occur. Having been through this myself, I am not questioning the desire for pain relief, I am questioning our methodology for pain relief at this point. The cervix will have completed the majority of this process by the time transition finishes and will then naturally rest while the uterus itself begins a nice contraction back around the baby. This is generally a pain free time and a great time to rest. It may take 15 minutes or a couple of hours, but there is often a period of rest here.

Mom now has time to adjust to the full cervical dilation, the feeling of the baby's head in that cervix, the further spreading of the ligaments through the entire pelvic floor. The intensity of contractions has subsided and will not pick up again until her body and the baby are ready for pushing/fetal ejection reflex. Unfortunately, it seems that this period of intensity is forgotten for what it is, and so many an epidural is given here with questionable use. If she is just about to have the relief she needs and requires full use of her muscles and faculties to push, why do we give an epidural now?

NOTE: We'll describe the process of epidural later, but know that this is not a quick and painless (or risk free) process itself.

Often times, I've been present at transition in birth where the pain is already wearing off for the mother, yet the epidural is just finally being inserted. The mother-to-be has weathered the pain on her own, and instead of being allowed to experience that natural rush of endorphins that is about to come and flood the entire body, she is given a medicine that will prevent her from using her legs and most often, from feeling what she needs to feel to push. Some nurses will check cervical dilation (incredibly uncomfortable and unnecessary and can lead to cervix stopping its process) and claim that transition has not started based on measurement.

Additionally, the process of measuring dilation is entirely subjective: practitioners insert their fingers until they can feel the cervix, and spread their fingers apart to assess the width of the cervix. Given the variation in human perception as well as finger width, it is ironic that dilation (a very subjective measurement) is considered such a strict measure of progression.

Transition is just a concept to describe physiological changes occurring on a spectrum. In the same way we cannot pinpoint cervical dilation as an indicator of progress (even beyond the subjectivity of measurement, a woman might spend a lot of time at one dilation and then speed along for the rest), to say transition begins absolutely at 8 (and a variable, personally defined eight at that!) is ludicrous.

SECOND STAGE

Once the cervix is fully dilated, contractions will tend to move further apart, have less intensity and the mother often has time to rest. The baby has moved downwards with this pressure on the cervix and its consequent opening and now the part of the uterus that rests just under the rib cage needs to shrink back down around the baby's buttocks/legs. The baby gets a moment of rest here too before the full and final descent through the birth canal. All too often this phase is either rushed or ignored and mom and baby DO NOT get the time for rest they need.

But the body is: 1. Not ready to push yet and 2. Needing rest. So, augmenting labor at this point by stimulating the uterus with either forced pushing or medication can contribute to postpartum hemorrhage.[44]

While a lot of the mainstream literature suggests that transition is followed by pushing, many feel that TOO little emphasis is given to this potential period of rest.

Generally speaking, women should not push until the urge to push is overwhelming. My own sense of pushing in the hospital paradigm (with the strict emphasis on continued management of labor) is that the reason many women say they felt no strong urge to push (outside of medication) is that they were not given the time to let their bodies rest before that strong urge came on and were asked instead to begin pushing well in advance of the 'right time'.

Additionally, within normal labor parameters, a woman should push with her own sense of the contractions:

> *"Don't resist what your body is doing; don't resist the pushing sensation if it is there. But as long as you can breathe with contractions and the pushing urge, there is no need to add extra pushing effort to what your uterus is doing. When the contraction holds your breath involuntarily, then add pushing technique to it."*[45]

As labor is completely individual, some women find that transition leads immediately into pushing. This, too, is normal. It is also less likely to concern the hospital staff, which is why I have spent the majority of this section discussing the longer process that also, and equally normally, often occurs.

In Chapter 6: Labor environment, we cover the fetal ejection reflex in more depth, but it is worth an overview now. Michel Odent speaks of this phenomenon that is only seen in uninterrupted births and generally not witnessed in a hospital setting; a phenomenon he says that is crucial to the labor process and the catalyst for he, himself, changing his labor and delivery methods in order to best promote it.

The name fetal ejection reflex, strangely scientific for such a profoundly organic process, comes from studies done by Niles Newton on the birth process in mice. Michel Odent later coined the term in regards the similar response in humans:

> *"An authentic fetus ejection reflex takes place when a human baby is born after a short series of irresistible contractions, which leave no room for voluntary movements. In such circumstances it is obvious that the neocortex (the part of the brain related to intellectual activities) is at rest and no longer in control of the archaic brain structures in charge of vital functions such as giving birth. During a fetus ejection reflex, women can find themselves in the most unexpected, bizarre, often mammalian, quadrupedal (on all fours) postures. At the very time of the birth and during the minutes following birth, at the beginning of the interaction with the newborn baby, these mothers seem to be in an ecstatic state."*[46]

The reason I bring this up here is that the whole concept of 'pushing' has become such an active and forced idea in our medical delivery model that we need to step back and understand just how reflexive this second stage of labor can be for mothers who are supported in an ideal labor environment.

Regardless how the mother experiences this second stage, whether active pushing or an ejection reflex, the second stage is the stage that baby is birth into the outside world.

DELIVERY OF THE PLACENTA

Once the baby has been born, the placenta (an organ made during gestation which has nourished the baby all this time) will need to come out as well. So long as there are no complications requiring a quick removal, the placenta should be allowed to come on its own time as well, generally 20-30 minutes after birth. The placenta will come out with a few natural contractions of the uterus that occur spontaneously.

Midwives and medical staff are very watchful during this time to ensure there are no signs of hemorrhaging. An important balance between observation and allowing mother and child to bond is key.

KEEPING MOM WARM during this time is also critical as it will facilitate the proper balancing of the hormones immediately post-birth and prevent any fight or flight response from hampering this natural change.

Evidence supports that waiting for the umbilical cord to STOP PULSING before clamping and cutting promotes optimal conditions for both mother and child.[47] Many midwives have long practiced this and many hospitals are beginning to take notice as well.

REVIEW

Labor is divided into stages more as a guideline rather than a hard-fast-fact:

- Stage 1: Early labor, Active labor, Transition
- Stage 2: Pushing, Birth
- Stage 3: Placenta Delivery

Whereas the three phases are helpful to understand labor, breaking it down further into centimeters of dilation can create a false concept of 'progress' or 'lack of progress' and creates a lot of unnecessary stress for the woman giving birth, the partners, and attendants present at birth.

Using these principles as ways to understand the process of labor is really all they should be used for.

Important ideas to keep in mind:

Pushing is generally a spontaneous urge and best done at a woman's own pace and rhythm. The general hospital method of counting during pushing has been shown to compromise the baby's oxygenation.[48]

Labor lengths vary. There is no true average and many healthy babies have been born to healthy mommas after 36 hour labors. Labors over 12 hours are often erroneously considered 'long' and subject to intervention under Active Management.

The amniotic fluid often does not break spontaneously until well into labor and is an important cushioning for baby throughout labor. Rupturing the membranes can facilitate labor when done correctly but is not without its own complications.

It is very rare that a woman's pelvis is actually too small for the baby to fit through. It is more the case that drugs and posterior facing babies are the cause of what is termed 'cephalo-pelvic disproportion' rather than actual size restrictions.

The position of the baby is very important and posterior facing babies lead to a higher rate of interventions, though there are many techniques and circumstances helpful for turning (and preventing) a posterior facing baby. Consult a craniosacral therapist, acupuncturist or chiropractor who specializes in the perinatal period for posterior facing and early detected breech babies.

The placenta should be allowed to birth on its own (in absence of complications) as well as the cord being left to pulse before cutting.

There is no average dilation in real labor. Remembering WHY active management of labor came into existence will help you to understand why a 1cm/hour expectation for cervical dilation is faulty and generally only achievable through augmentation. Women can go through several centimeters dilation in a matter of an hour as well as staying at a certain dilation for several hours without it being indicative of 'problems' or ineffective labor.

6

"The lack of disturbance associated with giving birth at home allows the full expression of the labouring woman's "ecstatic hormones". These four critical hormones – oxytocin, beta-endorphin, epinephrine/norepinephrine and prolactin – act to enhance ease, pleasure and safety for mother and baby in labour and birth, and also give mothers and newborn an optimal start to breastfeeding and bonding. Successful breastfeeding (which is more likely after homebirth) and mother-infant attachment give irreplaceable and life-long health advantages to both mother and baby." Sarah Buckley

THERE ARE REASONS the standard hospital environment cannot provide the optimal conditions for birth. But this is not to say a woman should not birth in the hospital. It is to say that as her birth partner, understanding why these optimal conditions are important and being able to realistically assess how to bring more optimization into the birth room is part of your role and should be part of your discussion together as a team.

Each woman is different. There are women, in the midst of large family gatherings who birth their children. There are those that want to birth unhindered in the woods. Each woman should have the option to choose what situation suits her best. The interesting thing is that many women, by nature of our indoor and less-cyclical lifestyles, no longer remember what creates conditions conducive to birth. Other times, women are limited by a sense of responsibility towards having family members or others present whom they would not ideally choose, but do not want to offend.

From observation by midwives and physicians focusing on unassisted birth such as Michel Odent, there are some generally accepted conditions that tend to be most optimal for birthing women. The reason is that these environments/conditions support the hormonal changes that must occur during labor in order to birth a child.

When we analyze this 'cocktail of hormones'[49], we discover that these conditions are those that also support orgasm. Ina May Gaskin, renowned midwife, explains it as the sphincter law as we mentioned earlier. Sphincters (the cervix, the anus, etc.) will not open when watched. The cervix, the muscle that opens to allow the baby to pass, needs to be safe and relaxed. So in the same way we need privacy for our most intimate functions (bowel movements, love making), so we need the same for birth.

For the most part, especially if a woman is more concerned about 'letting go' or releasing into the strong sensations (that can very much be orgasmic), the OPTIMAL CONDITIONS are:

Silence

Darkness

Warmth

Solitude/Support

Safety

& NO or MINIMAL interruptions

"*A laboring woman needs to feel protected against any stimulation of her neocortex (thinking brain). Since language is a specifically human stimulant of the 'big brain', this leads us to rediscover the importance of silence…Light is also a well-known stimulant of the neocortex. There is a well known 'darkness hormone' called melatonin. Our pineal gland releases this hormone at night to reduce the activity of our neocortex and fall asleep…It is noticeable that spontaneously, when women are not influenced by what they read or what they have been taught, they often find postures that tend to eliminate all visual stimulation, e.g. on all fours.*" [50]

Sarah Buckley, MD, in her book, *Gentle Birth Gentle Mothering*, describes the hormonal cocktail of labor: Oxytocin, Beta-Endorphin, Epinephrine/Norepinephrine, Prolactin:

OXYTOCIN: Engenders feelings of love and altruism, creates uterine contractions, aids in fetal ejection reflex and placental ejection reflex, responsible for euphoric feeling after a birth, leads to bonding of mother and child and let-down reflex in breastfeeding.

BETA-ENDORPHIN: Analgesic (pain relief), creates feelings of mutual dependency (bonding mother-child-father/partner), rises during pregnancy and increases throughout labor, helps women to transmute pain and enter levels of altered consciousness characteristic of undisturbed birth.

EPINEPHRINE/NOREPINEPHRINE: The combination known as catecholamines constitute our fight or flight mechanism. In the first stage of labor, where things can still be stopped in the face of danger, high levels can inhibit oxytocin production which consequently slows labor.

One mother's story:

"The familiar slow beginning of labor was underway. I felt the sensuous contractions that reached down into the nerves of the vagina. I've always felt like this is a referral from my cervix but I am not sure. My hips were loose, my heart felt full, and the tightening of my belly was unmistakable. Although two weeks before my due date, I knew it would only be a few more days and she would be here. But then we got the news. My father was threatening us with a lawsuit against our midwife. We suddenly had no labor support and an active attack against us. Everything stopped. There was no more sweet feeling, no more contractions and it took 5 more weeks before the situation had resolved to a point that allowed the baby to be born."

The catecholamines also increase again sharply at the end of birth in order to help mom do what she needs to do to get baby out (fetal ejection response) and help in the bonding of mother and child.

This is why, in earlier reference, and we will mention again, MOM NEEDS TO BE KEPT WARM AFTER BIRTH, so the hormones can rebalance. High catecholamine levels cause 'fight or flight' to stay in place, increasing risk of hemorrhage and decreasing bonding and lactation ability.

Baby's catecholamine levels are also necessarily high right at birth in order to be alert, breathe and take in new environment. However, they will also importantly and rapidly decline once in contact with mother and ready to relax back into lulled state.

PROLACTIN: Major hormone in breast milk synthesis and production and aids in the protective (mother tiger) effect.[51]

Fetal Ejection Reflex

There are some behaviors we no longer regularly see in labor, some elements I longed to discover for myself in the absence of any outside viewers. I know this is such an odd idea to so many, but I simply wanted to trust my body and surrender to the experience without anybody around me. I did not want the input of anyone else's sensations, feelings or potential judgment. I just wanted to find myself so I could birth my baby.

It was later, after I gave birth to my third child, that I read about the Fetal Ejection Reflex.

As mentioned in Chapter 5, the reflex only occurs in uninterrupted labor and is a quick series of involuntary contractions that birth the baby, rather than a long series (or hours) of pushes: *"In optimal physiological conditions, there is an obvious release of high levels of catecholamines during the very last contractions. A woman who may have been passive appears full of energy, moving into an upright position, looking for something to grasp, perhaps and becoming more vertical of bending forward. Potentially there is the sudden expression of fear with reference to death."*[52]

Odent's theories suggest that the neocortex (the linguistic, conscious part of the brain) can easily get in the way of our more primal reflexes. In my undergraduate studies in Anthropology, I was always fascinated by the birth experiences of Lisa!Kung woman. In this book she describes her solo birth experiences in the field. This was the way women birthed for a long time. Our bodies developed over years of evolution as primates and into our years as humans prior to such strong interference (from the neocortex, social brain) with our primal responses.

The thing about the fetal ejection reflex, or transition, or any part of birth that seems intense to the outside observer is that we tend to use these moments to try and reassure the woman. But in these instances, INSTEAD OF STEPPING IN WITH LANGUAGE TO REASSURE (and thereby completely interrupting the moment), WE NEED TO LET THE WOMAN BE.

"In other words, any interference tends to bring the laboring woman 'back down to earth' and tends to transform the fetus ejection reflex into a second stage of labor which involves voluntary movements."[53] Again another reason to follow the natural urge to push rather than force into pushing, which may not even be required.

We'll come back to the ways in which you can be present and when to step in during labor in Part II, but for now, keep this in mind: There are times in birth when silence and patience are the best strategies no matter how intense it may seem.

I found it so interesting that Odent also referred to the fact that it was not the moment of birth itself, but the moment when your child crawls up onto your chest and you spend your first breath together 'on the outside' that the CLIMAX of birth (the full culmination of all the intense pleasure/pain) occurs. I have both witnessed this at other's births and experienced this at my own and my reaction to his observation was "YESSSS!"

Though the availability of silence, darkness, support, warmth and safety can be increased in a hospital setting, there is one factor that cannot be prevented: interruptions. By nature of active management of care, nursing staff are required to monitor mother and child at regular intervals (fetal monitoring, cervical evaluations, etc.) The entire hospital environment is one of great interruption. We often feel that the trade-off in 'safety' (being in a hospital) is worth the interruptions though the evidence supports otherwise. And unfortunately, people CHRONICALLY UNDERESTIMATE the impact of all these interruptions.

For example, the fight or flight mechanism is constantly put into effect through monitoring and exams. This reflex is ONLY necessary at the very end of the labor as part of the fetal ejection reflex/pushing. The constant release of catecholamines during labor (due to continued interruptions) is very disruptive.

Making an analogy to something that might be more familiar, consider what it is like to sit on the toilet trying to have a bowel movement. Maybe you are at home and relatively comfortable with your partner outside the door, but say he/she comes in to get something. Many people automatically shut down and hold onto the bowel movement until the partner leaves. Imagine, now, this doesn't happen just once, but every time you are just starting to feel the great pleasure of release, your partner or now a complete stranger enters the room. Now imagine you are on a toilet, with no stall, in the middle of the room, being monitored. Because we have come to picture birth as this highly interventionist activity, we forget how very personal and rhythmic it is and do not apply the same principles to the birth environment that most of us would apply to our intimate spaces.

Activation of the fight or flight response is probably the least talked about but most important factor to consider in the opening of the cervix and the woman's ability to birth. <u>If there is reason for a mother to feel unsafe (whether physical, psychological or spiritual in nature), labor can be slowed or stopped altogether.</u>

Some common, often overlooked situations that can pose a 'threat' to a laboring woman:

- Change of circumstances (nursing shift changes, move from home to hospital, new people in the birthing room, lighting and noise changes, instrument sounds and monitoring).
- Physical interventions (IV's, Cervical exams, Fetal Heart Rate Monitoring, Blood Pressure Cuffs).
- Emotional Distress (Birth attendant stresses and concerns being transferred to the mother, mother's concerns over birth and transitions, history of trauma or negative pain experiences, abuse, etc.).

Though we often assume low risk births are acceptable at home while high risk births ought to take place in the hospital, there is evidence to show that even high risk birth becomes riskier with constant intervention.

Rixa Freeze comments:

"Although studies generally have compared groups of "low risk" women, some evidence suggests that home births might offer an advantage even to "high risk" situations. British statistician Marjorie Tew analyzed all births occurring in Great Britain,

categorizing them into various risk levels. She found that for every level of risk, except the highest for which there were not enough numbers to be statistically significant, hospital births had an "excess of deaths" compared to home births. This was true both for analyzing actual place of birth versus intended place of birth (in other words, still counting hospital transfers as home births). Tew's analysis suggests that birth outside of hospitals may have a protective effect even on women who are "high risk"—the ones always assumed to benefit from hospital care."[54]

The environmental needs for a laboring woman do not change just because she is considered high risk, yet the medical model tends to create an environment of fear and constant intervention that raises the stakes that much higher. This is not to say that a home birth is the only answer, it is to point out that no matter what the birth circumstance, high levels of interruption can create significant difficulties in labor.

The importance of the Freeze quote is that it suggests that it is the environment of uninterrupted birth that creates positive birth outcomes. Optimal labor environments are crucial to healthy deliveries.

7

INTERVENTIONS

"The humanization of birth does not represent a romantic return to the past, nor a devaluation of technology. Rather, it offers and ecological an sustainable pathway to the future." Ricardo Herbert Jones, OB

IT WOULD BE NICE to be able to say that interventions are only used as needed. But as the previous chapters should have highlighted, the medical model perceives birth as a problem needing constant intervention and aid, even when everything is going just fine. All too often, when couples are being told about an intervention that the hospital staff would like to begin, the information given is weighted towards the side of the need for intervention without adequate mention of the risks. Furthermore, many of these interventions are not discussed in the light of other options. An important aspect of functioning as a doula (in your role as advocate) is knowing the benefits and risks of the various procedures and being able to ask the staff about the reasons, having time to weigh the risks/benefits.

In the list below, I will review the risks associated with what are often taken as standard interventions:

Amniotomy (rupture of membranes)

- Does not reduce cesarian rate
- May increase non-reassuring fetal heart rate
- May increase rate of neonatal and maternal infection
- Can lead to umbilical cord prolapse

Electronic Fetal Monitoring (continuous)

- Increased likelihood of instrumental vaginal delivery and c-section does not reduce rates of stillbirth, low Apgar scores, or cerebral palsy

Elective Labor Induction

- Associated with increase in use of pain medication and epidurals
- Increased incidence of non-reassuring fetal heart rate patterns and shoulder dystocia
- Increased incidence of c-section and instrumental vaginal delivery

Epidural

- Triple a woman's chance of dying
- Result in temporary paralysis in every 1 of 500 cases and permanent in 1 of 500, 000
- Result in 15-20% chance of fever in mother which can lead to a host of interventions including a spinal tap on baby
- 10% of epidurals don't work at all
- 15-35% of women will suffer from urinary retention after birth
- 1/3 of women will suffer epidural-related back pain for days, weeks or months after birth
- Interfere with the mechanisms that guide the rotation of the baby as it descends through the birth canal, leading to sub-optimal

birthing positions (like posterior), resulting in more interventions, including cesarian section
- Lead to decreased oxygenation to baby in 8-12% of cases
- Decrease the sense of urgency to push as well as the ability to push

Episiotomy

- Does not improve neonatal outcomes
- Results in more pain, rectal tears, poor healing, weaker pelvic floor muscles and worsened sexual functioning

Cesarian Surgery

- Increased likelihood of infection, complications from anesthesia, surgical injury, hysterectomy, need for blood transfusion
- Chronic pain, breastfeeding failure, poor physical or mental health, infertility and life-threatening placental attachment problems in future pregnancies
- Increased risk in repeat c-sections

Immediate Cord Clamping

- Likened to a 'rather severe hemorrhage' for baby
- CONVERSELY: If the cord is left intact for a longer duration, this ensures immediate skin to skin contact on mother's warm belly immediate mother-child interaction, and helps to regulate the newborn's temperature and blood sugar levels, minimizing crying and helping to ensure successful breastfeeding.[55]

Pitocin

"Synthetic oxytocin [AKA PITOCIN] administered in labor does not act like the body's own oxytocin. First, syntocinon contractions are different from natural contractions, and these differences can cause a reduced blood flow to the baby. For example, waves can occur almost on top of each other when too high a dose of synthetic oxytocin is given, and it also causes the resting tone of the uterus to increase.

Second, oxytocin, synthetic or not, cannot cross from the body to the brain through the blood-brain barrier. This means that syntocinon, introduced into the body by injection or drip, does not act as the hormone of love. However, it does provide the hormonal system with negative feedback—that is, oxytocin receptors in the laboring woman's body detect high levels of oxytocin and signal the brain to reduce production. We know that women with syntocinon infusions are at higher risk of bleeding after the birth, because their own oxytocin production has been shut down. But we do not know the psychological effects of giving birth without the peak levels of oxytocin that nature prescribes for all mammalian species"[56]

Artificial Rupture of Membranes:

- Unless the cord is prolapsed or there are other signs of distress (immediate heart rate problems with baby or meconium in the fluid), women can be left up to 4 days without risk. However, we tend to force women to birth within a 12 hour window in current practice.
- Early rupture reduces baby's cushioning during the labor which can lead to increased fetal distress.

8

THE IMPORTANCE OF CHOICE

"Defensive medicine occurs when doctors order tests, procedures, or visits, or avoid high-risk patients or procedures, primarily (but not necessarily or solely) to reduce their exposure to malpractice liability. When physicians do extra tests or procedures primarily to reduce malpractice liability, they are practicing positive defensive medicine. When they avoid certain patients or procedures, they are practicing negative defensive medicine." Congressional Office of Technology Assessment

"In the process of [childbirth] becoming a matter for experts, the danger is that the real expert–the mother– loses her own right to knowledge and control." Ann Oakley

I HAVE SPENT so many chapters writing about the nature of our medical model and the inherent risks within this model because it is very difficult to make informed choice without all the data. But I hope the data only serves to broaden the picture that has been painted by our medical institutions rather than suggesting what a woman should choose. No matter my own personal ways of giving birth, my fundamental belief is that it is only the woman who can choose what she needs from her birth. Each woman's background, beliefs and needs are so different that to say there is 'one way' is ludicrous.

Most women do want to know the realities. Some would rather let others decide for them. But in either case, each woman is taking a certain type of responsibility.

It is important to know if the woman you are serving is wanting to take the responsibility for birth on herself and make informed decisions so you can advocate for those decisions.

It is equally important to know if the woman you are serving would like to leave these decisions in the hands of others (medical staff, midwife, etc.) so you can step back and let these external decisions be made.

Either way, you need to know where she stands so you can support what she chooses.

If you find yourself disagreeing with her decisions, you need to talk.

If she is not choosing what feels right to you, consider carefully what this really means. Do you feel she is lacking in adequate details? Or do you feel like you just know better?

Who is giving birth? Can you possibly know what situation is right for her?

These questions are not easy and this can be a very tough road to walk.

I have seen women who wanted hospital births and husbands who wanted home births as well as the reverse and so many shades of grey in between even if it is often times the husbands who are more in line with the medical paradigm. Much has been written about why, including the overall more masculine sense of wanting to 'fix' things (occurs in men and woman) since the medical model follows more closely in line with this idea of 'fixing'.

What is not considered as often is how being on the 'outside' of birth makes it impossible to really know what is going on on the 'inside'.

What this means—and this will become more apparent as we speak about 'techniques' and ways of being in birth—is that stepping in and trying to fix often feels better to the partnered or less embodied persons (the ones NOT giving birth) in the birthing room because the internal experience has not been available.

This does not only apply to men. I have met many a mother and female physician or nurse in the delivery room who sees birth as something painful to be fixed and who cannot envision birth in any other paradigm. That is part of the travesty of our medical model and the years of distancing women from their own process.

SO, here is the hard part:

A woman, ideally, has all the information she needs to make her decision.

She makes her decision from the place she is currently at in her life.

This decision may or may not resonate with you.

Depending on your relationship with this woman (is she your wife, daughter, best friend?) the level of discussion about the expected birth experience will vary.

But in the end, HOW she decides to birth is HER CHOICE and a doula/partner must support that choice fully. The same release of catecholamines (fight or flight response) that occurs with interventions and unsafe circumstances in birth also has a high chance of occurring when the support staff is fearful or antagonistic towards the woman birthing. If you are in the birth room, or a strong presence in this woman's life throughout her pregnancy, your negative views, emotions and potential lack of support can go a long way towards impeding the birth process. A woman is necessarily open and receptive during pregnancy and in birth in a way that can also leave her differently equipped to keep these negative external forces at bay.

Keep this in mind.

Though you are helping to advocate for her choices in a medical or midwifery environment, you are NOT responsible for making the medical decisions themselves. You do not have to know everything about birth. You need to TRUST this woman and to TRUST the process of birth (or trust that the practitioners are well-versed in birth so that you can portray calmness and trust of the process itself).

Ideally, you just need to support her where it is right for your partner.

One mother I was a doula for had done all the research she could, decided that she wanted an un-medicated birth and hope to avoid c-section at all cost. Towards the end of pregnancy, however, she began to have some concerns about the child. As her doula, I was also having intense premonitions about bad outcomes. I even called both the head of the hospital's family birth center and one of my trusted midwife colleagues to discuss with the nature of premonitions in birth and how they handled them in their practices. Everything in me wanted to tell the mother to go ahead with the planned c-section. But instead, we discussed all the options available and what she was feeling. This mother went on to call upon all of her trusted resources to ask about their experiences in birth and get the information she needed to make her choice. In the end, she did decide to do a scheduled c-section, even though nothing else suggested she should, and baby came out fine, though the OB did indicate later that there were physical signs that the birth may have been problematic.

Another mother I worked with was having a very good progression in her first labor. I had my hands on her back for much of the early first stage in order to help her with the pain she was experiencing and I could feel the baby descending nicely. The mom had indicated in our pre-labor interviews that she was concerned about her pain threshold and said she would likely seek an epidural but just wanted to labor as long as possible prior to pain relief. At the point that labor really began to intensify, the mother decided she was ready for the epidural. Given that she had barely reached 4cm and not a long ways into labor, I had concerns about the impact this would have on her labor. As a doula, I brought up the information we had spoken about earlier (how an epidural can sometimes slow labor) so that she remembered the risks because information like this is easy to get lost in the labor-mind of a woman giving birth. She said she knew the potential risk but did not feel like she could handle the pain becoming any more intense and did not want to try any other methods for pain relief (position changes, etc.) She had been very scared going into labor and the fear had really not subsided. She went ahead with the epidural, and even though it was hard to see how the epidural did slow and change the nature of her labor, it was my job to support her choice and work with her in this new set of circumstances. Nobody knows what the outcome would be either way. This was HER labor.

Trust in the mother's inherent wisdom–in what she knows about her own body and process–is what is required of everyone attending a birth in order to properly serve the birthing woman.

The paradigms for mother-friendly childbirth developed by The Coalition For Improving Maternity Services (CIMS) are well worth considering @ www.motherfriendly.org

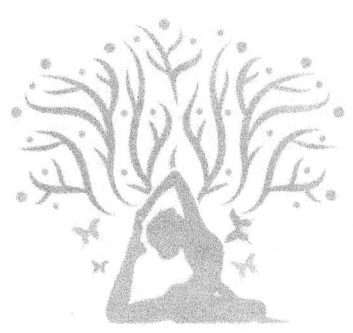

PART II: BEING A DOULA

9

"MMOC (Midwifery model of care) practitioners are not afraid of labor pain or of watching women experience it; they know that their own calmness facilitates the woman's ability to move through the pain without producing the anxiety that increases it." Robbie Davis-Floyd

L ABOR IS A DANCE. The mother-to-be and child within are responding to cues in one another and to the messages also from the external world. The interplay of hormones, emotions and physical changes manifest as the wisdom of RHYTHM. Like a couples dance routine, we can break down the physical movements and give a 'technical' overview (Phases of Labor), but what really determines the outcome is the 'artistic' component. Each mother and child—if the

52

circumstances are right and the mother is allowed to sink into the dance—WILL FIND a unique rhythm and flow that is exactly right for that particular labor.

The general rule of thumb for doulas:

When the mother and child find their rhythm and flow,

we don't interrupt.

Instead, we HOLD SPACE.

The process of labor has been designed to bring babies into this world in an effective manner. Mother and child work synchronously. With the right conditions (generally darkness, relative solitude and silence, and safety) a mother will find her own way to birth.

To 'Hold Space' is the most profound skill a doula, or any person, can develop. Not only will this skill help you be a strong, supportive partner in labor, it will give you the ability to sit with many people and any situation with grace.

Holding space is the art of simultaneously being yourself while putting the needs of another at the forefront and giving complete love and acceptance. This does not mean you have to understand what that other person is going through and it doesn't mean you might not feel afraid. Holding space does not mean you have all the answers. Holding space really means you are willing to sit in the space you are in without running away, turning away or having to control it.

It is like holding the space in front of you and all around you as though it is one big open vessel. And in that vessel is everything that is happening in the labor. And in that vessel is your commitment to hope, light and a positive outcome.

For those of you who have meditated or practiced some form of yoga or martial arts, holding space is similar to the state you enter when focusing on the breath and movement.

Holding Space is the PRESENCE you have in each moment. During birth, this looks like PRESENCE amidst UNCERTAINTY while creating a feeling of TRUST and SECURITY.

EXERCISE IN HOLDING SPACE

Sit still in the midst of a busy space, whether at home around others or out in public at a cafe or park. Notice how your body feels. Just take stock. Are you relaxed, tense? Notice your emotions. Are you upset, joyful? Notice your thoughts. Do you feel this is a waste of time, a curious event? Now let yourself drift past even these ideas and sensations, aware of your state of being without necessarily trying to change it, and feel out into the room around you.

What do you notice about the room itself? Is it warm, cold, welcoming, hostile? Try to get a quick sense of each person in your immediate environment. Notice whether these people are tense, happy, concerned, carefree, etc. Look at what they are wearing, notice the expressions on their faces, get a sense of how it feels to be sitting here in your own state of being while feeling and watching other people's states of being.

Now, see what happens when you project certain states of being into the room. Let's say you simply sit with a frown on your face. Pick something that makes you angry and let it really be present in your body for a moment. Now look back out into the room and see how it feels and looks to you. Has anything changed?

Let's choose the opposite sensation. Choose something that makes you feel incredibly joyful. Let that really become a part of you. Allow yourself to smile and become that joy. When you feel like you are full of joy, look back out into the room and the people around you and see what you notice.

Our states of being impact others and vice versa. We are impacted by the states of being of others.

In the delivery room, there will be MANY different states of being in each of the professional and personal members present. You are not there to change their states of being, but you are there to notice their states of being and your own. You are there to assess the dynamics in the room and provide an effective barrier for your partner, a loving, open, caring space where she can dive deep into the process of birthing no matter what is going on in the room around her.

Think of it as creating a bubble that does not prevent her interaction with the outside world, but mitigates it.

Where you are in your space at home now, or at the park or cafe, wherever you are, choose someone you notice who seems to be struggling somewhat. Now, assess your own state of being once again. Take a few deep breaths and let yourself feel grounded, centered, and at home in whatever mood you are in, and then create a large circle or bubble that encompasses you and this other person you have chosen.

Let yourself feel feelings of empathy, warmth, generosity and care for this stranger. Allow yourself to take nice deep breaths and exhale calmness into the space you share. Do this for 2-3 minutes.

Now look around the space you are in and notice how the room feels. Notice how others appear. Notice how the person you are focusing on is behaving, responding, changing with your focus. You do not have to stare at them while you do this. You can simply be very aware of where they are and allow them into this shared space through attention.

Finally, see if you can get a sense, just by letting your thoughts and feelings drift, as to what this person is feeling now. Do you think they are more calm? More stressed? We are not trying to prove that you can read another person's mind here, we are just practicing the very real ability we each have to feel another person's state of being. How we interpret it is another story. The KEY in holding space is to acknowledge you are feeling SOMETHING from this person and then to let even that go. Let them feel how they feel, let their state of being be just fine. Allow yourself to feel comfortable with however they are feeling and just keep breathing and centering yourself in your own body.

Send out a sentiment of wellbeing, of generosity and care to the entire room now and then close that connection with the room down, come back entirely to yourself and simply notice what you feel, what you are thinking, what this experience has taught you.

I would encourage you to practice this daily. It only takes 5-10 minutes per day to really engage. You can do it anywhere, in the elevator, on the bus, in a dance club, at the gym.

Even 1-2 minutes gives you enough time to get a sense of a room and your place in it.

Holding Space — being aware and present with your state of being and the states of being of those in the delivery room, including and especially your partner—allows you to create a safe, supportive and caring environment for the woman in labor that she will feel and respond to. In labor, our bodies are SO sensitive to everything going on around us and when at least one person puts their full trust and care into us, that makes ALL the difference in the world.

10

"The first line of care for minor delays and complications is with low-tech interventions such as position changes, emotional support, massage, immersion in warm water, aromatherapy, herbs, homeopathy, hand maneuvers and most fundamentally, 'changing the energy' by working to create a more positive and trust-based atmosphere; higher-tech interventions are reserved for cases of true need." Birth Models That Work

B E PRESENT, hold a warm, open, supportive space in which the birthing woman can find her own rhythm and voice, so she can ask for what she needs and know you are there for her in whatever her needs may be.

The #1 Main Technique is Holding Space (Chapter 9)!

This is, quite seriously, the SINGLE MOST important thing you can do and should not be underestimated.

As everything leading up to this point indicates, a woman in labor is a formidable force full of wisdom and needs mostly to be allowed to find her own way through the labyrinth of birth.

All the rest is certainly helpful when you work together, but nothing compares to your willingness to maintain a presence of calm, open acceptance.

HOW DO YOU KNOW WHEN TO STEP IN AND BE MORE ACTIVE?

1. When she asks you.

A woman in labor can seem like the weather: very prone to quick changes and extreme conditions. This is natural and to be expected. She is trying to figure out what works for her and it is an amazing gift to get to be a part of this. Listen closely to what she is asking. Follow her requests. They might change quickly as she navigates the rapid changes occurring within her. Just go with it. Whatever it is she needs, try to meet. She is giving you trust and speaking deep wisdom even if it feels chaotic to you. The more you listen and respond, the more she knows you are there for her and she knows you trust in her abilities. Let yourself be a blank slate in this regard. Let yourself be a part of her transformation and this incredible ritual.

2. When she seems to be moving away from the plan you talked about in advance of labor.

What is discussed prior to labor is completely up for grabs during labor once a woman is inside the deep changes that are occurring in her body. That does not mean she wants to go against what she said in your discussions, it simply means, she has all this new information to contend with that she didn't have in advance and her mind is in a very different state.

If you have ever pushed yourself to the limit to stay up for several days at a time or finished a marathon or done other rituals that would take you into an altered state of being, you might be able to have a glimmer of the type of mindset a woman enters in labor. It is altered in the best of ways. But she is also highly suggestive and seeking a path through the intense sensations she is feeling.

So, it should come as no surprise that she might ask for things (ex. pain medication) that she said she did not want in advance of labor. This is completely normal and frankly to be expected. Your job is not to tell her yes or no but to remind her that she had certain intentions that you had talked about before. Make your words SIMPLE. Sit with non-judgement. And still, BE YOU.

Ex: "I cannot even imagine how you are feeling right now. I understand you want an epidural. Would you like to try turning on your other side first to see if that feels better?"

3. When someone else on the team is moving away from the plans you made together prior to birth.

It is absolutely a time to speak to the other health care providers when they are suggesting interventions or options you know your partner was not interested in. Get the information. Know that you have time to decide together. Find out more from the team what their reasons are. Let them know what your partner's wishes are. You are her advocate. Talk with her. Tell her what is being considered. Discuss together. You can wait to speak with her in between contractions. Allow her time to consider the information she is being given.

The is often the sense of rush in hospitals that is not felt at home births. It can be very difficult to determine what is a forced rush and what is truly emergent. But use your skills in assessing others. Think about how you assess those you work with or for or those that work for you. How do you determine when they are telling the truth? When there is something else going on? When you know you are only getting half the story? All these same skills apply in the birth room. Put them to use. Dive in and figure out what is really going on.

Ask the staff direct questions such as: "When does this decision need to be made?" "What are the risks and benefits?" "What can we do to help my partner birth the way she feels is right for her?"

4. When your gut tells you to step in.

Go with your feelings as well. If you see that your partner is struggling and you do not feel like you are projecting your expectations onto her, then ask. Ask her if she needs you. It is good to ask specific questions like: "Would you like ice to chew?" "Would you like a warm or cool cloth on the back of your neck?" Would you like me to put pressure on your low back?" She might not know what sounds good until you say it and she might not be in a state where she can conceptualize exactly what she needs. So open ended questions like "what do you need?" can be too confusing to receive a clear answer. But yes/no questions (Do you want a cold compress on your forehead?) are easier for her to integrate into her changing body state. In that moment, it either sounds good or it doesn't.

TOUCH

Some women love it, others hate it. Some will flip flop. It may take awhile to figure out what touch she is looking for. Sometimes this means having a hand on her shoulder, holding her hand, holding her feet. Sometimes this is holding her head or curling up in bed with her to hold her entirely. Likely, each moment will bring a different need. One minute the pressure is too much, the next it is not enough. This is the nature of childbirth!

Touch can be comforting, such as curling up in bed with her when she is in a restful state and needing to feel someone close. Or simply a hand on her leg to let her know you are there. Notice how she responds to your touch. Whether she is relaxing into it or resisting. If you are not sure, use your yes/no questions: Is my hand here good? She might say yes, she might say move it over here or she might say to get your hand off of her. Either way, you will know and that is perfect!

Here is one example of comfort touch. One hand on her forehead, one hand on her heart, her body weight leaning into you. This can be soothing, supportive and restful.

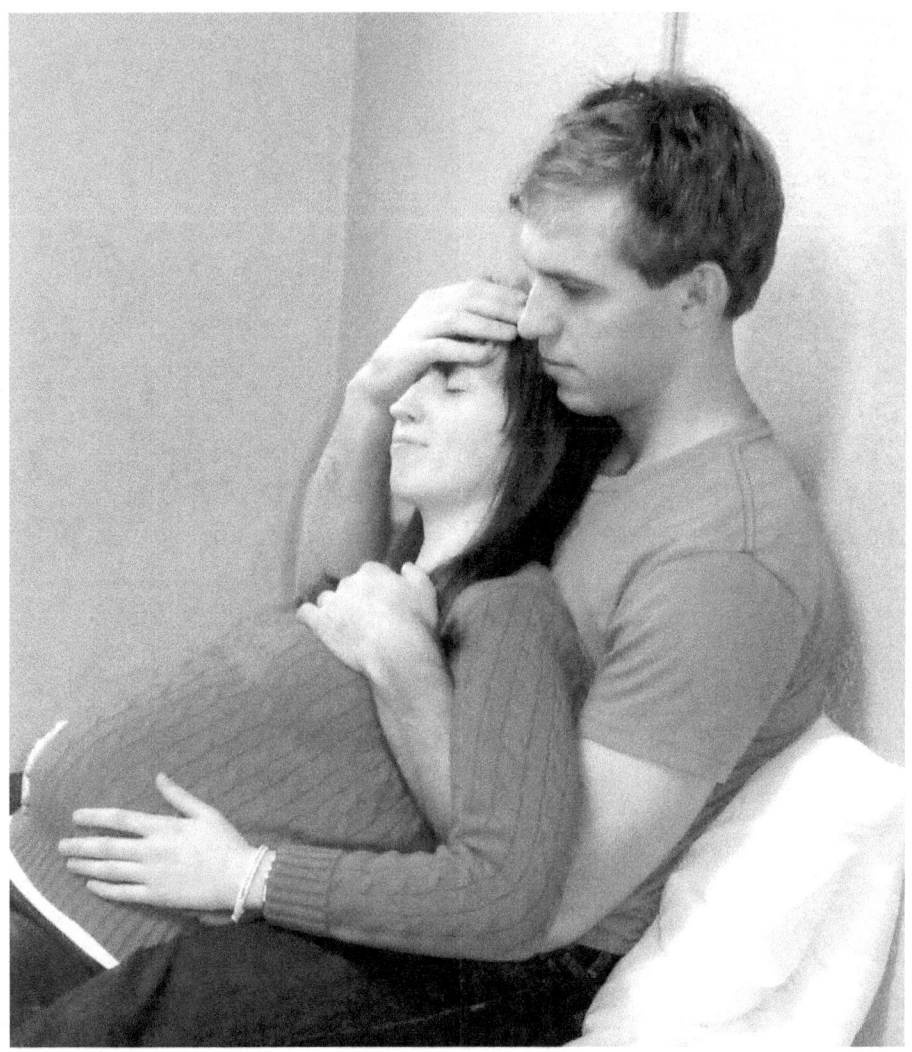

Another example of comfort and grounding touch, just holding her ankles.

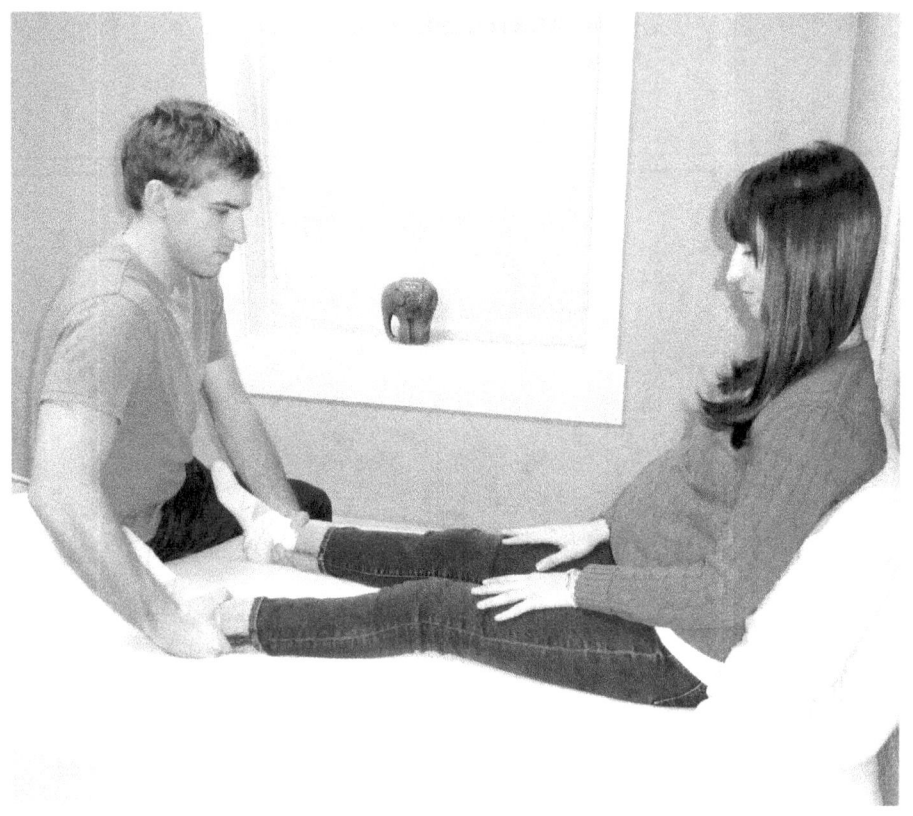

Touch can reduce the pain in specific areas as well.

The double hip squeeze can take the pressure off the sacrum, off the low back and provide relief as the pelvis opens with the baby's descent.

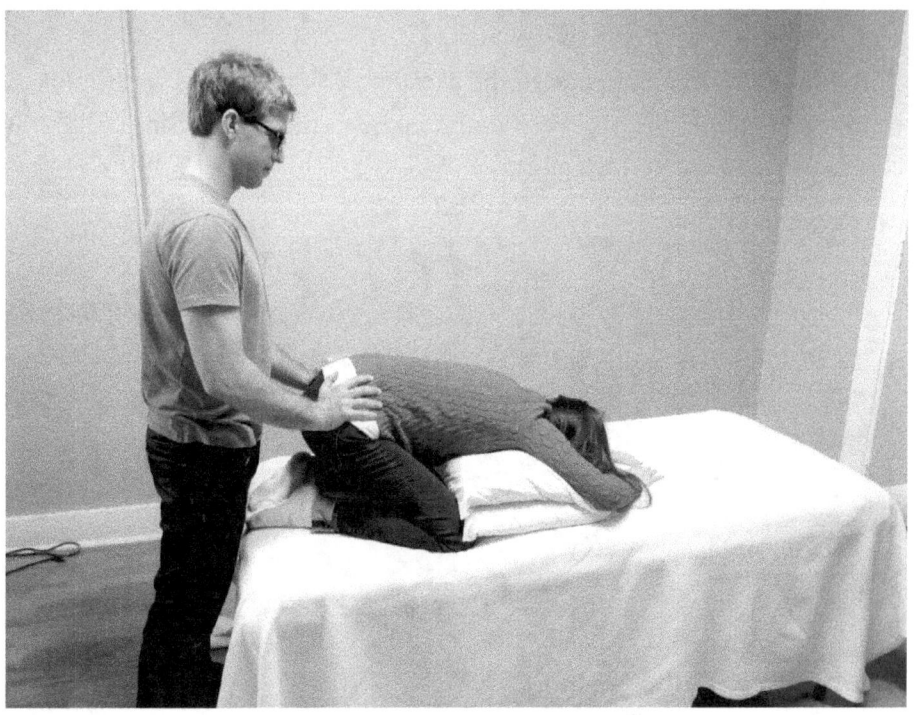

To do: Place each hand to either side of the sacrum and lean in with your body weight as much as she would like. You might find yourself leaning in quite far and be surprised at how much pressure she can take. Trust her.

Pressure points to either side of the sacrum. You can use your thumbs to relieve pressure at the low back and help open the pelvis. Similarly, you can use fists to create pressure.

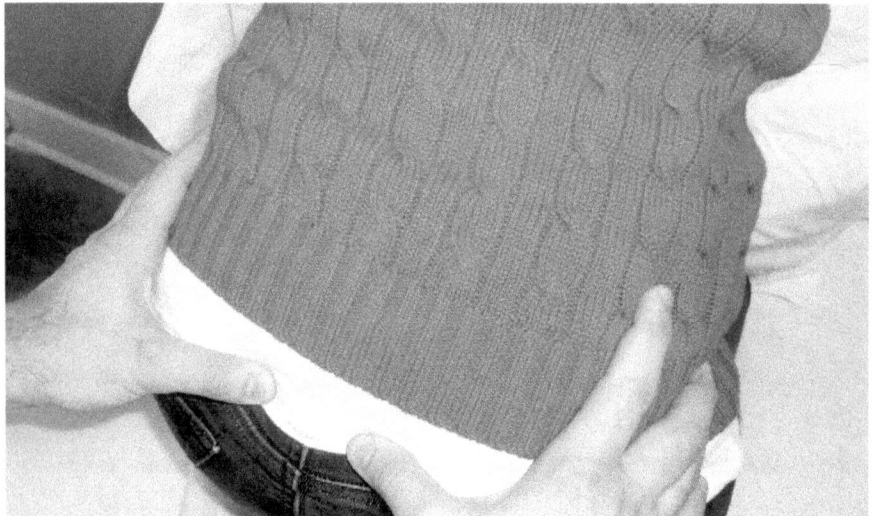

A double hand on the sacrum itself can relieve the immense pressure of baby's head moving down further into the pelvis. No matter what position mom is in (all fours, leaning forward, side-lying) you can provide this counter pressure.

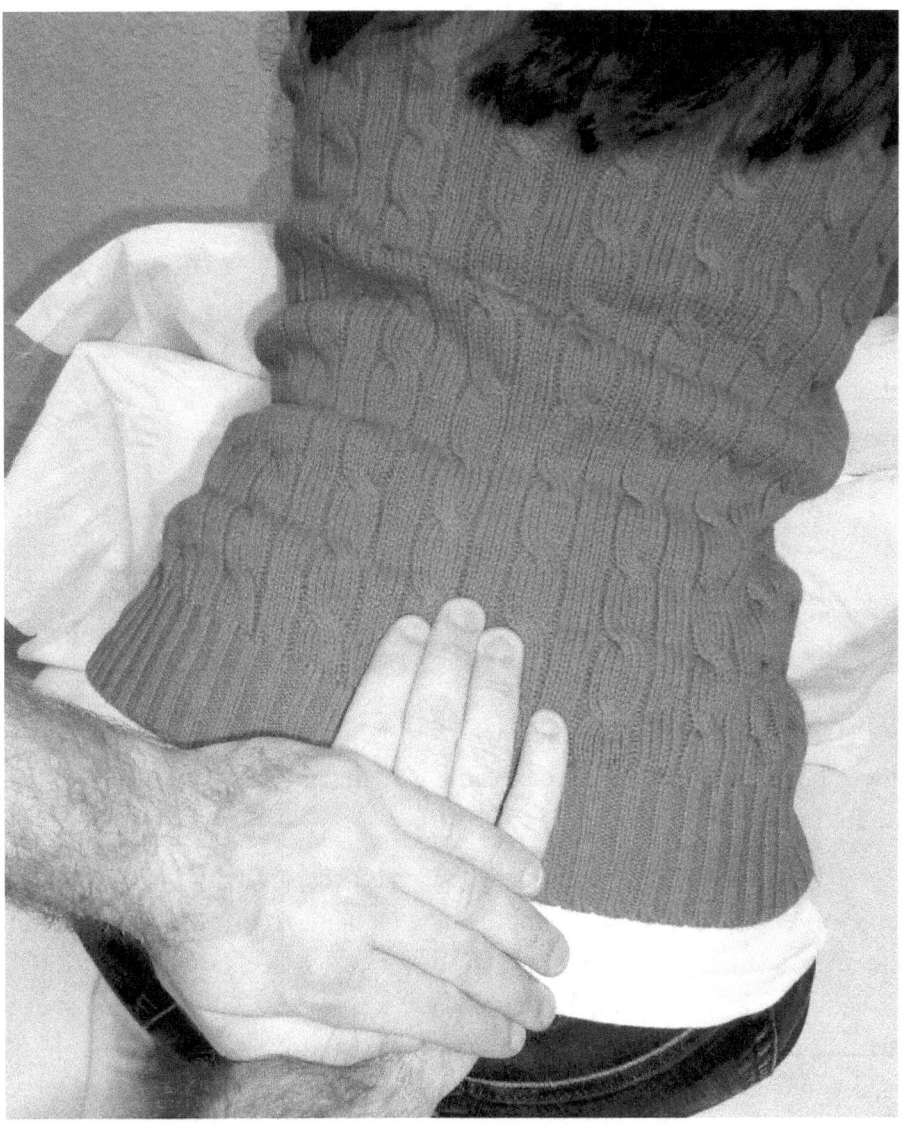

This double handed pressure allows her to acclimate to the intense sensations and feel grounded, and like there is some barrier on the pain. Something she can push against.

A lot of time is often spent in this position.

But remember, it only works if it is working for mom. So, if your partner does not like it, it isn't helping.

CHANGING POSITIONS

One of the key elements of birth is movement.

If mom can walk and squat and dance and sway and move, she is not only helping to alleviate the pain, she is helping to bring baby into this world. All these moments and the power of gravity combined create the right conditions for baby to birth.

Keep in mind, however, two things:

1. Because movement helps bring baby, some positions will cause the sensations to be more intense.
2. Most of us no longer spend our days on our feet or squatting and developing the strength and comfort that these positions use to bring.

Because of this, women who thought they would love to spend their labor walking sometimes find that the intensity of walking and squatting is more than they expected.

If you can help mom find a way to keep moving with rest and support and breaks to lie down, that is excellent. **Remind her that these positions are bringing the baby closer.** This is a powerful psychological statement that gives her purpose for the intensity she is feeling and reminds her she is not wandering around only in a world of intensity but that her movements and willingness to birth are actually bringing forth a baby; that her efforts are worth it!

If you are walking and her contractions come on strongly, she will likely want to lean on you. This is wonderful.

Let her put her arms around you and lean into you and move and squat and sway as she needs to allow the contraction to work its way through her body and do the work of birthing.

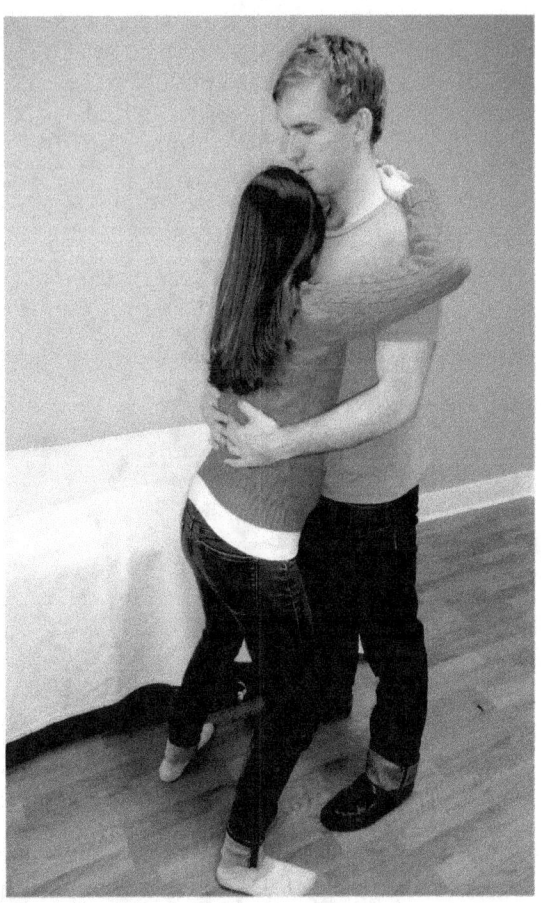

Allowing your partner to rest against you while up walking or simply to rest against you staying still in a room gives her the support she might need during contractions while allowing gravity and the opening of her pelvis to work with the baby's movements.

Similarly, you can support the laboring mother by sitting on the edge of a bed or up against a wall and allowing her weight to sink into you with her back to you and your arms holding beneath her arms.

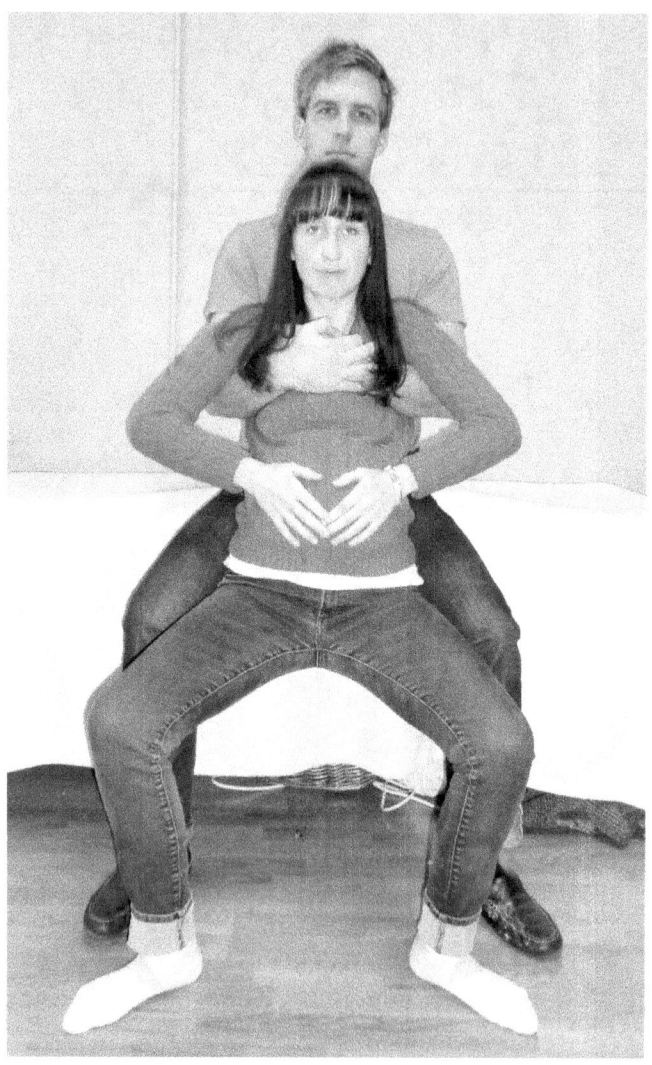

Even when not up walking or standing, the birthing woman can change positions in bed. Below we see her sidelying. She may also want to be on all fours, swaying and rocking through her hips.

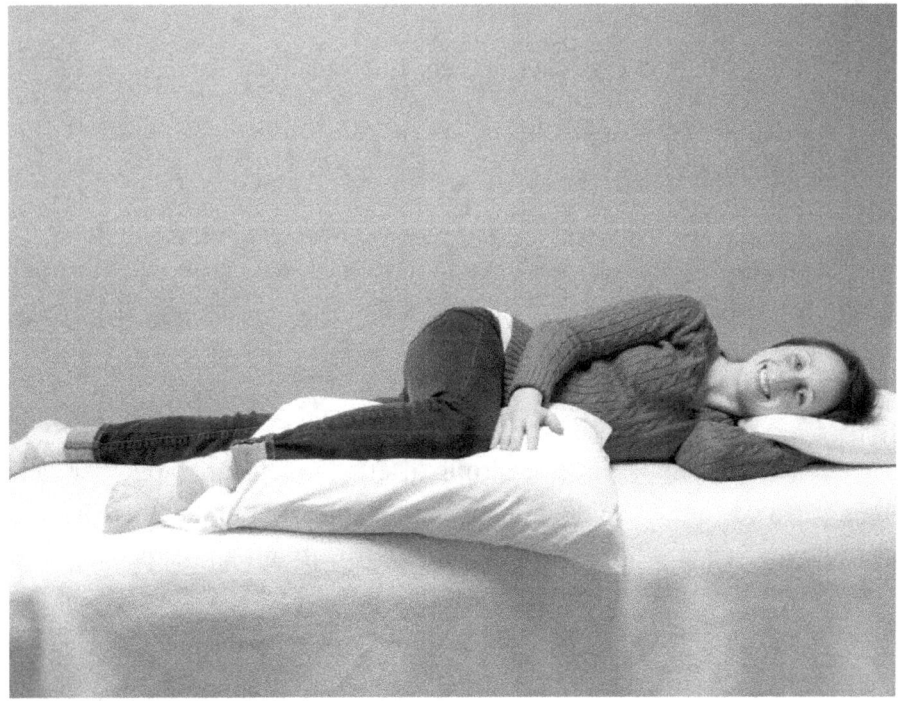

I hesitate to give a list as though there is any one position that works for everyone, but in today's world, we don't spend much time squatting and our muscles are not generally strong enough to squat through an entire labor. However, squatting affords the maximum movement and gravity for baby to emerge, so if mom can squat part of the time, it is a good position.

Some positions make labor more intense. This is what we want. That means labor is progressing. However, that can feel like too much at times. If so, give encouraging reminders that each contraction/surge brings the baby closer to this world. Breathing down into the pain is another useful technique. Sometimes the sensations are intense and a woman may want to avoid that intensity. This is understandable. But there is also a point where the birthing woman realizes that the intensity is productive. You can help her by continuing to frame contractions and intensity as positive aspects of baby coming closer.

BREATH

In birth as in every other facet of life, breathing is KEY.

This doesn't mean you have to know any advanced Yogic Breathing, however.

The key is to remind the birthing mother to breathe. And more so, to breathe deeply yourself. We respond to the world around us through entrainment. And when a birthing mother's team is breathing deeply and staying centered in their own bodies, the mom will also follow suit.

Breathe WITH her.

As contractions come on strong offer: "Let's breathe together" and then proceed to breathe deep long breaths into your abdomen. She will follow your example if you keep breathing without any expectation or judgement. These are just reminders that it is possible. That breathing is possible even when in pain. The breathing INTO the intensity, in fact, is helpful. It gives her control she might sometimes forget she has.

NAUSEA

Ginger teas, staying hydrated and nourished (especially when she is still feeling like eating in the early stages) and electrolyte solutions are all excellent ways to minimize nausea. Remember, vomiting can be an excellent way to clear some room, as well, so it is not the end of the world if mom pukes during labor! It is when the nausea is strong for long periods of time or the vomiting does not stop that it is of concern, mainly for fluid loss and when it becomes a focus for the birthing woman.

One of the key factors is for mom to be eating well in general and staying hydrated prior to the birth. Keeping the body balanced and consuming small snacks and fluid when labor begins as well. This helps to give her the nutrients she needs (again think of running a marathon) over the long haul.

It is important, in general, to offer sips of water throughout labor and to have electrolyte solutions on hand (whether commercial or homemade). And if ginger is something she likes, it is helpful with nausea, so keeping ginger tea in a thermos or ginger-ale on hand or even ginger lozenges to suck on.

This pressure point can be helpful for nausea. Hold for one minute at a time with a one minute break repeatedly during waves of nausea:

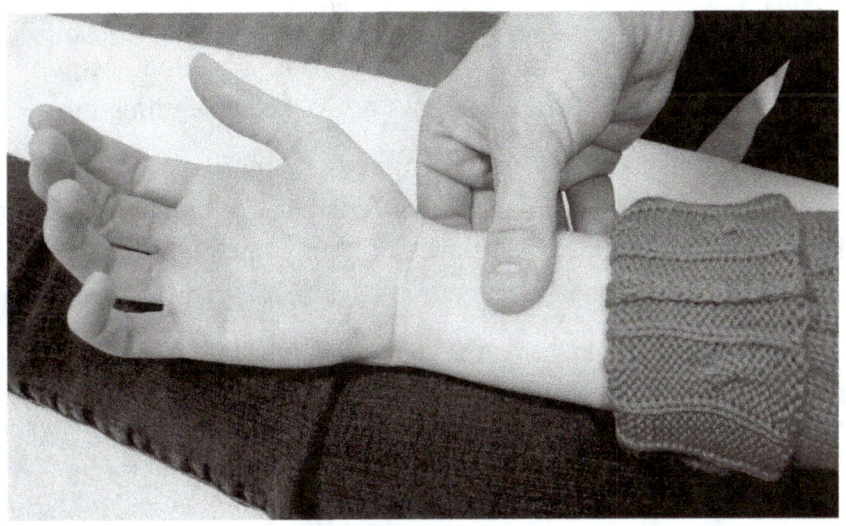

HYDROTHERAPY

Using warm or cold cloths. Forehead, neck (usually cool) and warm cloths at lower abdomen just above the pubic bone. Eases the tension on the muscles. Can feel wonderful. Ask simple questions: Warm cloth on your forehead? No. Okay. Cold cloth? Ok. Let's try it.

Baths. Especially later in labor when mom needs a rest, baths can be very calming, allowing the cervix to continue to open but giving her body needed relief in the buoyancy. Placing a towel over the belly and pouring water from a cup over the belly continuously can be very soothing.

Showers. A shower is another great relief for some women.

If the place you are birthing offers water birth, this is yet another wonderful option.

SOUNDS

Keeping sounds to a minimum from the outside world and keeping disruptions at bay is part of the ideal set of circumstances we talked about in earlier chapters on optimal birthing conditions. But just as there is no one right way for anything, some women love to have things moving and going around them. So, follow mom's lead.

But if you think she is just trying to be nice and accommodate people, see if you can arrange to have things kept at a minimum.

Music, like touch, can be soothing one moment and aggravating the next. Have music on hand for different stages in labor. Sometimes the sounds are ones in which she can find rhythm, other times, they are a welcome distraction, and sometimes, again, it is just too much input.

Either way, if you have music on hand, it becomes an option during labor, so it is worth bringing into the birth environment.

ESSENTIAL OILS

For many women, mint and ginger are helpful with nausea and lavender can be soothing. Bringing oils into the delivery room to have available to sniff from the bottle works and if mom wants to put some behind her ears then she can do so.

THINGS TO KNOW FOR THE STAGES OF LABOR

Labor is an ongoing process with no clear delineations between the phases and every woman labors differently. Still, having some sense of how a woman is feeling and interacting at various stages of labor is necessary for you to know as her doula/partner support.

Early labor

Important for mom to continue eating if she feels like it and taking in fluids. Protein rich and nutrient dense foods are best.

Walking and going about daily activities- allows labor to progress but keeps mind on other things

Mom may want you to be with her or she may want to be alone. Follow her lead. Assure that you are there when she needs you rather than hovering if she doesn't want you there.

Moms are generally excited in this time. Labor has finally begun and is warming into the body.

When she feels like resting, encourage rest. This may be a nice time for a massage to the legs, hips, back and shoulders. (Inset for massage) Benefits

If you are going to the hospital, have things ready to go.

More intense labor

Speak clearly, close up. Offer succinct choices 'water or juice'. The laboring mother is focusing inwards ever more so and is in a completely different world than the one you are inhabiting. She may make demands for what she wants or may struggle to figure out what she wants. Either way, take nothing personally. She is finding her rhythm and making her way deep inside to prepare to open wide enough and draw out her raw energies to birth the baby.

Very intense labor

The breakdown

Take NOTHING personally.

She is literally in an altered state. Speak clearly. Yes/No questions.

After baby arrives

Once baby arrives, be with mom (and baby both). Tend to her needs still.

KEEP HER WARM.

There will be a lot of cleaning up and flurry of activities going on. As much as you can stay with mom and baby, do.

Keep her hydrated.

Provide as much stillness as you can for her in terms of holding space in stillness amidst the busy flurry of activity. Remember, just your ability to hold a calm presence alone will change her perception of the entire room.

There are important reasons moms are watched during this phase (most specifically, this is the time the medical team watches for hemorrhage and placental delivery).

Still it is very important for mom to continue to feel supported.

I like to say that after the baby is born, the mother gets born.

And most women identify with that idea.

We go through a huge shift in hormones, sensations, etc and identity. Nearly ten months pregnant and bonding internally, here our child is suddenly outside of our body and as excited as we might be to have come to this point, there is invariably a sense of loss that is either conscious or subconscious, but a very natural part of the process.

Now that labor is 'over' in most of the professional team's eyes, it is easy to forget that the mother is still laboring in different ways and so it is not in fact finished until sometime after baby is born. Sometime well into that first year.

As her doula/partner, you can preserve sanctity of space.

Hold her literally or in holding space, keep her warm, hydrated, full of love and support. Make sure she is able to get rest.

74

Ask for interruptions to be minimized, etc.

Mom not only has to now learn how to care for this baby outside of her body, but how to care for herself as a mother.

Your biggest gift now can be understanding this fact.

11

DOULA SELF-PREPARATION

1.Take a deep breath everything is going to be okay.

This is a comment for YOU, not the mother. What you feel is translated to what mother feels. Pregnancy and labor give the mother the ability to sense the world around her much more acutely. This is an incredible skill that makes her much more able to care for the infant in utero as well as follow the cues of labor, but it means each and every interaction with a mother in these periods is heightened.

If you already follow a practice of meditation or conscious thought, use it now. If you do not, it is not hard to do it only takes a willingness to do it. The idea is simply to take a breath, let go of your worries and be right there in the moment with the mother.

Keep breathing.

2. Consider your own ideas about birth and pregnancy

Take a minute to write your thoughts about birth and pregnancy on a sheet of paper. Write out your fears and hopes. Write anything that comes to mind. Now is not the time to censor.

Read it back to yourself. What do you notice? Where are your fears? Where might you limit the mother's possibilities by holding onto these fears?

What do you need to do to set them aside?

3. Receive body and/or energy work

You are going to provide nurturing touch for the mother in labor and throughout pregnancy if you are a direct part, and it helps to understand the importance of this sacred space even if you are not directly involved. By receiving body and/or energy work, you learn to tune into your own body and can better understand what you are transmitting to the mother through your touch and intentions whether up close or at a distance. Your own increased self-awareness is of great benefit to the mother.

4. You cannot know what she is feeling and that is okay

Every woman births and gestates differently. If you are not a woman or you have not gone through birth and labor, it is not necessarily something you will understand through your own body and experience. Even if you have, your experience may be worlds apart from hers. THIS IS MORE THAN OKAY. The mother does not need you to identify with what she is going through, rather she needs you to be there with her and help in the ways she asks for without any pretense that you know what she is going through. Most people, in general, do not like to be told: 'I know exactly how you are feeling'. But we all respond positively to the comment: "I am here for you."

5.Take care of yourself

Counter-intuitive as this often sounds, this is incredibly important during pregnancy and labor both. If you are not eating and sleeping well, getting exercise and tending to the things that bring you joy, you will quickly deplete yourself of the ability to be present for the mother.

During labor, it is easy to forget to eat and drink, but you must. Your strength and stability are important resources for the mother. Make a point to take these breaks and be clear that you are leaving for 15 minutes to eat and will return promptly. Keep a water bottle on hand for your own self and small snacks like nuts and granola bars that you can eat quickly in the room that bring you energy and sustenance.

6.Take another deep breath and keep on breathing.

Your job is not to read the cues of the labor and pregnancy and determine potential problems and risks. Your job is to hold the belief that everything is going to be just fine so the mother can sink into her body and wisdom in a safe and secure environment that breathes nurture and love.

12

Over the course of this booklet, these ideas of support, advocacy and trust have been woven throughout the overall message, but it is worth pointing them out individually and highlighting the importance of this trio.

SUPPORT:

Your support of the birthing mother is critical. What you do and how you behave prior to birth, during birth and after birth has a significant impact on the mother-to-be/new mother.

At other times during her life, what other people do may have less impact, but during labor especially, and also during the hormonal, emotional, psychological and spiritual transformations that occur throughout pregnancy and beyond, a woman tends to be much more impacted by the views of others, especially those they love and respect.

No matter how much you learn or how much you believe you know, the reality is that you are not inside of her body and you cannot know what is the best way for this mother to birth or to be.

What you do know, what you can demonstrate at all times, is that your support makes all the difference in the world.

Your support creates an atmosphere of trust, safety and respect and a space for her innate wisdom to flourish.

ADVOCACY:

Advocacy is the process of taking the support for someone and acting or speaking on their behalf, or supporting them in acting and speaking on their own behalf.

Advocating for someone is not assuming what they want or not. To advocate for and with someone, you need to be continually checking in with that person to find out what it really is they DO want or need.

In terms of birth and labor, having a dialogue prior to birthing and during labor is what will allow you to advocate for your partner. Whether this is asking for more blankets, having a doctor explain a procedure until all facets are understood or asking another family member to leave the room when they are not wanted, these are all forms of showing support for your partner, for speaking when she cannot or standing by her so she feels strong and capable of speaking.

TRUST:

You must trust her and she must trust you.

How does she trust you? When she knows you trust her.

It really is that simple.

When you put your full trust into her ability to birth this child, it does not mean you expect her to do it all herself or not ask for help or to know what she is doing at all times, it means that you trust that she will figure it out, will work through it, is more than capable of undergoing this transformation. It means that you RECOGNIZE the IMMENSITY of the TRANSFORMATION she is undergoing and realize that it is its own process and wisdom that goes far beyond you.

Trust on this level does not mean you are not aware of the fact that there can be problems in labor. There are times a person needs more outside help. There is the very real fact of life and uncertainty. Of course.

But you are also trusting the process of birth. This process that is not perfect but is exquisitely designed to work on more levels than just bringing forth a child. This process works to create bonding between mother and child, to induce lactation, to empower the mother for the long term care of her child and to teach her things about herself she needs to know for the years to come.

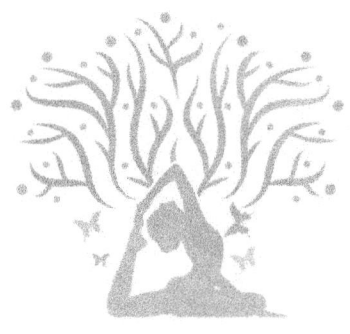

PART III: POST PARTUM CARE

15

As is probably clear by now, birthing a baby is just the beginning of another journey.

Mom is busy birthing herself now as well.

Making plans for after the birth is an important aspect of preparing for birth. Make sure to talk through your family's postpartum needs for privacy, nourishment, rest and support.

For some women, having plenty of family on hand will be ideal. For many others, too many visitors, even family, is more stressful than helpful.

In some cultures, the woman and child are on bed rest for at least the first week if not longer, kept warm, fed restorative meals and attended to in all ways. In this way, mom gathers her strength, sinks into to the breastfeeding process and bonds intensely with child.

Of course, your own situation will determine how you are able to approach postpartum, but in a society so consumed by the lead up to birth, the active process of labor and the notion that a woman should just return to her 'normal' self in no time at all, we have forgotten both the very sacred nature of bonding and healing postbirth and expect mothers to be something they are not: they are not who they were before.

Even if you can prepare to have the first 3-4 days postpartum as mom's 'lying in' days where she and baby are alone together in the bed and attended, this is an amazing beginning for the whole family.

If you are the person who will attend to mom, talk to her about what she will need and make these arrangements in advance.

Ex. Have casseroles cooked and frozen, easily available for you to cook. Or, even better, create a meal train or have someone who wants to help create a meal train (see below). Have all the baby supplies ready and in her bedroom. Learn to massage or hire a therapist to come give mom a massage (if she wants this). Arrange for limited family visit times, or ask everyone to wait until after the first week to visit. Keep a freezer bag full of maxi pads soaked in witch hazel for vaginal healing (see below).

Whatever your list of things to have ready, be prepared not only for the birth itself but for the very necessary down time after birth. A time of quiet, of rest, of good meals and of bonding.

Go easy on yourself and go easy on mom.

Experienced marathon runners know they need to prepare for their recovery time in order to stay healthy and strong. Birth is no different.

Some things to have ready for postpartum (beyond the diapers, etc.):

MEAL TRAIN: One person arranges for the community of friends and family to deliver home cooked meals (as per mom and family's dietary needs) for the first 1-2 weeks postpartum. Meals are delivered on a schedule and people understand this is not a time for visiting. Visiting will come later.

PRECOOKED MEALS FROZEN: If you have the space, cook meals in advance that can easily be frozen and then rewarmed. Cook healthy, nutritious meals that will restore mom's energy, iron levels and support milk flow. This is to say, high protein, good fats and plenty of vegetables.

FROZEN MAXI PADS: Lay out 14 long length maxipads. Pour at least 5 tablespoons of witch hazel onto each one, enough to soak the cotton pad. Place on a pan in the freezer for 30 minutes. Remove pan and place maxi pads into a large freezer bag to keep frozen until needed individually. These are invaluable healing aids post vaginal delivery.

MOM's FAVORITE SNACKS: Have some high nutritional value snacks on hand like nuts and seeds, homemade power bars, and plenty of water at mom's bedside so she can easily snack and stay hydrated throughout the day without having to leave the room.

BOOKS, BOOKS ON TAPE, MOVIES, MUSIC: Have some forms of easy entertainment on hand so mom can sink into them if she decides during her bed rest.

MASSAGE: You can learn the basics of swedish massage for free here: http://introswedish.weebly.com Keeping mom's back and shoulders stress and tension free is HUGE after birth. She has done so much work this past ten months carrying a baby and whether she delivers vaginally or by cesarian, her body has been through an immense amount of work and change. The more she can be touched and loved in soothing ways on a daily basis, the better (if this appeals to her). Even 20 minutes each day works wonders and increases your bonding time together as well. Consider also bringing in a professional therapist who focuses on postnatal massage or craniosacral therapy, or a similarly suited chiropractor to help with restorative therapies.

SANCTUARY: Create a sanctuary in the bedroom. Candles, wraps, etc. Have mom make it a space that will soothe and nurture her postpartum or put together the plans for how this will look so that you or someone else can prepare the room for her. For some couples, snuggling together postpartum is just what the doctor ordered and for others, having separate sleeping places (mom and baby in one bed and partner in another location) is the more restorative option. Discuss in advance. Discuss again once baby is born. If you are the partner, do not take offense if you are asked to sleep in a different location. This does not mean you will not and cannot have bonding time with baby. It mostly means that your sleep with likely be much deeper! Seriously, though, this is a crucial time and mom will know best what is best for her own recovery.

Creating a sanctuary also includes keeping mom free of stress or worry. Making sure other children are cared for and prepared for this transition. Limiting visits to short duration or altogether entirely (but being the one who runs interference and makes sure 5 minutes really is five minutes).

PLACENTA ENCAPSULATION: I understand the idea of the placenta alone is enough to make most people squeamish, but the benefits of cooking, dehydrating and then grinding the product into a fine powder for capsules that the mother will consume is incredibly beneficial for restoring hormone balance, improving and stabilizing mood, supporting milk flow, replenishing iron and other key nutrients that are depleted through pregnancy and birth and is also beneficial for baby. Many people provide this service or you can prepare to do it for mom by watching this video: http://placentacap.weebly.com

All in all, the way a mother is cared for is the way she is able to care for her child. The more care and support she receives, the more she has to give back. But moreover, because we start to think of mom as only mom and no longer an individual, we forget just how much care she really needs JUST FOR HER, just because she too is human and has worked incredibly hard and needs recovery period.

Sleep, nutrition, hydration and support. These are the fundamental needs a woman has in the postpartum period.

If you are available to be the primary diaper changer and food fetcher, house cleaner etc. for the first few days, fantastic. If you can designate someone to take care of these tasks, terrific. If it is a family member, make sure they understand their role. It takes a lot of energy to be responsible for visiting and directing someone's actions, and that is not what the mother should now have to do. Choose someone who can be of help and stay out of the way otherwise. A postnatal doula is another great option.

Finally, don't be alarmed at the large number of emotions the new mom will experience. It is one thing to read about it, and quite another to go through — for both of you.

There is no one way, no one right process, and the more you can simply be there to hold, to listen, to love and to learn, the more she is able to experience the broad range of emotions associated with birth and post-birth.

She is still very open to the emotions and interactions going on around her, so creating a stable, safe, warm sanctuary where she knows she is fully supported is the best way to give back to the mother who has already given so much of herself to creating, birthing and now nurturing a child.

QUICK GUIDE

For easy reference during labor

EARLY LABOR:

Mom is still able to talk and move but might need to stop occasionally for contractions.

DOULA TO DO:

Make sure you have the things you need ready for the hospital/home birth.

Encourage mom to take a walk, continue to go about her day and eat and drink at regular intervals.

Encourage mom to rest when she feels she needs to.

Time a few contractions so you have a sense of where things are at (the length the contraction lasts as well as the amount of time between contractions).

Listen, laugh together, remember and remind that this is all normal.

Stay calm, breathe, be excited.

If mom is feeling at all nervous, breathe together, walk outside, try some massage or just snuggle.

MORE ACTIVE LABOR:

Mom is not talking through contractions and they are getting closer together.

<u>DOULA TO DO</u>:

Time the contractions (between them and length of them). Keep note. Follow the plan you established with your doctor or midwife (to call when contractions get to a certain point).

Have mom continue taking sips of water or juice between contractions.

Allow mom the quiet time she needs to breathe through contractions. Be there for her to lean into you as she needs.

Make arrangements for childcare, transport, etc.

ACTIVE LABOR:

Contractions are intense and relatively close together and you are either in hospital or with midwife.

<u>DOULA TO DO</u>:

Stay calm. Hold space.

Follow mom's cues. Give pressure to her low back or hips if she is in pain.

Offer walking, changing of positions.

Ask simple yes or no questions.

Offer ice chips and ways to stay hydrated.

Encourage her to rest in between contractions. Compliment her on how well she is doing.

Rest with her.

Apply pressure to hips and sacrum while during contractions, let her move, vocalize and work her way through the contraction however suits her.

TRANSITION:

It seems like the world is ending.

She might be yelling intensely, suddenly super agitated and not at all certain about what is happening to her, she might feel like she is going to die or suddenly wish she would die.

<u>DOULA TO DO:</u>

STAY CALM. THIS IS NORMAL.

Focus on the here and now.

Help her focus on each contraction. Breathing into it.

If there is time in between contractions, encourage her to rest, compliment her on how well she is doing. Remind her everything is alright.

REMEMBER: Transition does not last that long but is often the most intense time. If you keep this in mind, you can help her remember too.

PUSHING:

She has the sudden urge to push or is encouraged to do so by the medical professionals.

<u>DOULA TO DO:</u>

Help hold her legs in position if she is lying down or support her if she is standing or kneeling.

Encourage rest and hydration between pushes.

Follow her rhythm and support her pushing rhythm.

CROWNING:

This means baby's head can be seen at the vaginal opening with each push.

DOULA TO DO:

Let mom know you see baby's head!

She will understand how close she is and find renewed energy.

Offer that she might feel baby's head or a mirror to see.

Continue to support her rest time between contractions/pushing.

Continue to support her body (legs, arms, etc.) as needed to assist in pushing.

Stay in rhythm together.

POSTBIRTH:

Baby is born. Placenta may or may not be delivered yet.

DOULA TO DO:

Ask for additional warm blankets. Stay with mom and baby.

Offer buffer between the busyness of the room and her experience.

Remember she is in an entirely new part of the birth process now and she still needs your immense support.

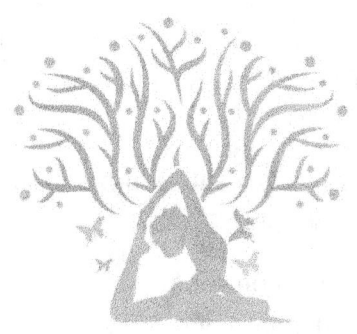

Visit www.goddessworks.me

I believe childbirth is inherently safe with some recognizable risks.

I believe environments that support uninterrupted childbirth and give the mother the ability to find her own rhythms are the most suited to a safe & empowering birth.

I believe that to look only at 'safety' in birth is to remove some of the most fundamental and transformative elements of birth that create empowered mothers and peaceful beginnings on this earth.

I believe birth itself has been removed from the hands and bodies of women and put into a technological world where others give the illusion of 'control' and 'safety', when, in fact, no one can perfectly assure a safe birth.

I believe, moreover, that the further away from our own bodies we move, the more the risks of childbirth are increased and the less we trust ourselves in all facets of life.

I believe lack of authority over our own bodies is the number one fear factor in our society as a whole.

I believe that by putting the control of our health in the hands of others, we have essentially denied our own capabilities, powers and responsibilities in our own health.

I believe health care providers are at our service and should be viewed as consultants rather than experts.

I believe that the ability to perform a c-section safely is a great benefit when needed.

I believe all women see birth differently.

I believe a woman is the one who should make decisions about her own body.

I believe that only a woman in her own body knows her own body and nobody else can tell her what she is feeling, or what she should do with that body.

I believe a woman and a child together in utero are the only ones who can make the decisions that will impact them both.

I believe whatever a woman chooses is up to her and should be respected REGARDLESS.

I believe EVERY WOMAN HAS THE RIGHT TO CHOOSE THE BIRTH SHE DESIRES.

I believe that KNOWING the realities of our birthing system is ESSENTIAL to being able to TRULY CHOOSE THE RIGHT OPTION FOR ONESELF.

I believe birth is transformative on every possible level. When we treat birth as sacred, we create a safe, nurturing and supportive environment for mother and child to thrive.

References

These are all excellent books with in depth information.

Baldwin, Rahima. *Special Delivery*

Block, Jennifer. *Pushed: The Painful Truth About Childbirth & Modern Maternity Care*

Buckley, Sarah, MD. *Gentle Birth Gentle Mothering*

Davis, Elizabeth. *Heart and Hands: A Midwife's Guide To Pregnancy and Birth, 5th ed*

Davis-Floyd, Robbie. *Birth As An American Rite of Passage*

Davis-Floyd, Barclay and Tritten, Eds. *Birth Models That Work*

Freeze, Rixa. *Unassisted Birth (PhD Thesis)*

Goer, Henci. *The Thinking Woman's Guide to Birth*

Hrdy, Sarah Blaffer. *Mother Nature*

Odent, Michel. *Functions of the Orgasm*

Rooks, Judith Pence. *Midwifery and Childbirth in America*

Sjoo, Monica and Barbara Mor. *The Great Cosmic Mother: Rediscovering the Religion of the Earth*

Wagner, Marsden, MD. *Born in the USA: How a Broken Maternity System Must Be Fixed to Put Woman and Children First*

ENDNOTES

[1] Wagner, Floyd, McCourt

[2] http://www.cdc.gov/nccdphp/publications/aag/pdf/drh.pdf

[3] http://www.cdc.gov/nchs/data/databriefs/db09.pdf

[4] World Health Organization. Appropriate technology for birth. Lancet 1985; 2 (8452): 436-7

[5] http://www.cdc.gov/nchs/data/nvsr/nvsr60/nvsr60_02.pdf

[6] http://abcnews.go.com/Health/section-rates-vary-widely-hospitals-study-finds/story?id=18656847

[7] Block, Jennifer

[8] R. Silver et al., "Maternal Morbidity Associated with Multiple Repeat Cesarean Deliveries," Obstetrics & Gynecology 107, no. 6 (2006): 1226– 32.

[9] http://www2.cfpc.ca/local/user/files/%7BCB26B78C-E421-4510-A76E-BA338489A90D%7D/CS%20US%20Meneker%20%20and%20Declerque.pdf (303)

[10] http://www.ncbi.nlm.nih.gov/pubmed/1635490

[11] Nissen E, Uvnäs-Moberg K, Svensson K, Stock S, Widstrom AM, Winberg J. Different patterns of oxytocin, prolactin but not cortisol release during breastfeeding in women delivered by caesarean section or by the vaginal route. Early Human Development 1996; 45: 103-18.

[12] Wagner, Richard

[13] Ibid

[14] Ibid

[15] Ibid

[16] http://www.childbirthconnection.org/pdfs/LTMII_report.pdf

[17] Davis-Floyd, Robbie et al. Birth Models that Work, Part One: Large Scale Systems. In this book, the authors give an in depth exploration of the statistical and socio-cultural components at play in the midwifery model of care for not only the Netherlands, but for many nations around the world who are demonstrating models of care more effective that the United States.

[18] http://www.motherfriendly.org/MFCI

[19] Rooks, Judith Pence, Midwifery and Childbirth in America, Temple University Press, p 465

[20] http://www.motherfriendly.org/Resources/Documents/MFCI_english.pdf

[21] Hrdy, Sarah Blaffer, Mother Nature

[22] Odent, Michel, The Function of the Orgasm

[23] Sjoo, Monica & Barbara Mor, The Great Cosmic Mother

[24] http://davis-floyd.com/birth-and-the-big-bad-wolf-an-evolutionary-perspective/

[25] Wagner, 100

[26] Freeze, Rixa, Unassisted Birth, 12

[27] Numerous sources repeat this information. Look to the books in reference section. All in depth explanations of how and why we got to now. And current books, Wagner and Block, speaking to the nature of our obstetric system and need for control.

[28] Davis-Floyd, Robbie, Birth Rites

[29] Ibid

[30] Wagner, Block and many other sources.

[31] Block, Jennifer

[32] Block pg 20

[33] Ibid, 21

[34] Wagner, 53

[35] Ibid

[36] Wagner

[37] Wagner, Block, Vincent

[38] Floyd, Wagner, Block

[39] Davis-Floyd, 111

[40] Freeze, Rixa, 199

[41] Davis-Floyd

[42] Davis-Floyd 139

[43] Davis, Elizabeth, Heart and Hands

[44] Ibid, 114

[45] Baldwin, Rahima, Special Delivery. 65

[46] Odent, 9

[47] https://www.rcog.org.uk/en/news/rcog-release-timing-of-clamping-the-umbilical-cord-analysed-in-new-opinion-paper/

[48] Goer, Henci, The Thinking Woman's Guide to a Better Birth, 97

[49] Buckley, Odent

[50] Odent, 10

[51] motherandchildhealth.com

[52] Odent, 13

[53] Odent, 12

[54] Freeze, 210-1

[55] Block, 25

[56] Odent